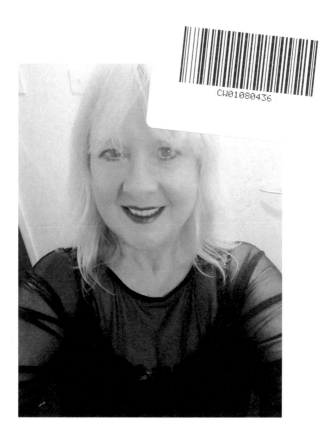

Carol Watson founded Rainbow Path Meditation Series in 2004. She has developed more than 200 guided meditation scripts to aid in healing, finding balance, bringing in peace, joy and wellness to her mentees. Carol facilitates online classes in Edinburgh, Scotland, and in-person. She is an accredited UK clinical hypnotherapist, life coach and NLP facilitator. She moved from a successful career of 22 years in print media into a holistic vocation which began with meditation and energy healing work and developed MA=RaY Light and S.I.R, Past Life Regression, adding complementary therapies such as reflexology, massage, sound medicine, then hypnotherapy, life coaching ad NLP into her life work.

Acknowledgements

Christine Sinclair, my meditation teacher and guide in Adelaide, Australia in 2004, who supported me in my spiritual development and growth, encouraging me to take the stand, so to speak, and run a class in her absence. Thank you for the confidence you had in me, my vision and voice, and my blossoming work. I am truly grateful.

To my mum and to my sisters, Lorraine, Maureen and Wendy, who have always been inspiring and magical, as we would talk about all things spiritual. For keeping the child-like wonder very much alive in me.

To Poppy Evans, and Anne-Marie Birch, my longest standing mentees in the circle over the years and wonderful supporters and friends.

To Nicola (Haynes) Tillbrook, for your constant belief in all the spiritual things I do. For absolutely just 'getting me'. Period.

Lorraine White, Calmblue Clinic, Edinburgh, for understanding what my work is all about and supporting me through the clinic to grow. You have been so pivotal in my success. Thank you.
To each of my attendees/friends who have journeyed within themselves during a period of time with me in the Rainbow Path Circles. I appreciate and value each and every one of you. Thank you to those beautiful tribe members who shared their visions or experiences within these pages.

To Great Mother, Great Spirit Mother/Father God, all the Ascended Masters, Archangels, Spirit, Animal Guides, and all who have come through my meditations to share their light and wisdom.

Stephanie Jeffery, my proof reader, sub-editor, and lovely friend. Thank you for bringing your insights and your knowledge to this wonderful project along with your unwavering faith and belief in it.

Carol Watson

Love-'LIFE' Meditations

Recovering Self by Re-mastering MY Life

AUSTIN MACAULEY PUBLISHERS™

LONDON ∗ CAMBRIDGE ∗ NEW YORK ∗ SHARJAH

A CIP catalogue record for this title is available from the British Library.

ISBN 9781398454347 (Paperback)
ISBN 9781398454361 (ePub e-book)
ISBN 9781398454354 (Audiobook)

www.austinmacauley.com

First Published 2022
Austin Macauley Publishers Ltd®
1 Canada Square
Canary Wharf
London
E14 5AA

Foreword
By Jackie Evenes

Let me introduce myself first, then I can offer you a preview of what you are about to venture into, through these magical pages. My name is Jackie Evenes, and as a single parent with two now mostly grown up children, I have studiously worked my way through a multitude of life challenges for what feels like decades now! I see these as landmarks of my own personal endurance and growth. I acknowledge my efforts and do try and salute myself on how far I've come.

So often we are somewhat too harsh on ourselves and don't take the time to congratulate ourselves for all the small victories as well the as bigger achievements we have made. I know I have come a long way and am grateful for all the good that has come into my life, including Carol Watson, who has helped transform my inner world and assisted me to evolve into the 'light-being', whilst still acknowledging the 'dark-side' of myself, I am. She is a great mentor and teacher.

I have come to 'Be'. Yes, just 'be'. I like where I'm at these days. I like me! With the support of the Rainbow Path Meditation Circle for more than a decade and a half, I have grown and stretched beyond all imaginings. I am happy to say I am now a qualified Yoga Teacher and Manage a beautiful holistic Studio, besides having two really great children that have also come a long way. I am very proud of them both.

So, let me share about the Rainbow Path Meditation Circle. Carol, who has a way of bringing laughter into the circle, a light-heartedness that is contagious and makes each individual in the circle, whatever circle she is running, feel at liberty to just 'be themselves' and to explore their inner landscape. This freedom of expression in a space that feels safe, allows the circle to share very intimate and personal things that enhance good listening skills and a strong sense of love, empathy and compassion within the group.

There is a strong opportunity for building one's capacity in storytelling skills; an age-old craft. As this naturally develops, the marvel of unique and collective colourings arise from the volume of amazing guided meditations that Carol has created over the years. I believe there are over one hundred and eighty meditations to date in her repertoire. That excites me, as I have experienced some fantastic ones in all the years that I have been attending Carol's classes, and there always seems to be something new to discover, whether it's a first-time journey or a revisit into a previous guided landscape.

There is an energy, an essence, which is purely the spirit of the amazing— 'Rainbow Path Meditation Series'. Even although you, the lovely reader, will most likely not be attending Carol's classes in person, you could online, (maybe you will if drawn), the solo journeying through these beautiful little gem stories could find you being part of the over-riding spirit of Carol and all of us, who have benefited beyond words, from Carol's joyful guidance.

You will meet aspects of yourself you never knew even existed, such as in the Yin and Yang balancing, inner journey. You get to see your own inner male and inner female self, who will show themselves in form, within your mind that is incredible. You then can decipher who is out-of-sync and who is over-dominant, within. It is healing! Recognising this is how you address this imbalance and be-friend these inner parts of yourself, making you actually feel more self-connected and complete. You begin to understand what needs attention and healing to bring you into wholeness.

The journeys focus on inner alchemy and external manifestation work; there are beings along the way you get to meet and work with such as your animal guide, or an archangel such as Michael, the Protector of all living beings. This is one truly magnificent guided meditation, and the psychic protection I feel with Michael and his Legion of Foot Soldiers is something I call upon all the time. It has been a life gift to me. To know your boundary or auric space is secure and protected is truly a real-life gift.

You will discover 'heavenly colours' on the colour journeys, as is the case in The Rainbow Ribbons, which in my opinion is both healing as well as truly magical. You'll be wise to find a gorgeous little diary because you will want to record some of the visions and feelings that you have after doing one of these amazing meditations. As Carol says, "it uplifts you when down to revisit the experience and read the messages that you get from those we connect with, in particular journeys." I agree 100%.

Carol also encouraged us all to get our creative juices flowing during the horrible global Corona Virus Pandemic of 2020, as we attended the circle weekly, online. The creations that were produced were so wonderful to see and kept us all going. You may see some of these creations throughout the book along with Carol's paintings she did in watercolour.

You will not only learn how to get in touch with your own self and aspects of yourself, guides and helpers, but you learn to breathe properly and deeply. Most people, certainly from time to time, will shallow breathe, or have a particular holding pattern, and so it's helpful to hold a deep full breath and follow with a conscious steady, natural smooth release as you read through these meditations as we do at the start of the sessions online or in-person. This cleanses a lot of the build-up of toxins from you and helps bring you into a more grounded and settled place. It enables you to experience better as it acts as a gateway to a calmer, mindful space.

We always connect heart-to-heart each time we meet, even if it is online and that is just beautiful. Feel it as you read the meditations. Stop and connect with us all on a puff of love, as we will acknowledge you, too. We feel the Rainbow Tribe connection with the extended circles too and that is warming for the soul, so be open to us all. During meditation, we make sure to bring those loved ones into our Pillar of Light sending them all love support and healing if they choose to receive. It is all a matter of choice and as Carol says, "We are not here to affect anyone's karma. If someone wants to experience any discomfort or painful lessons then it is their choice."

So I wish you a beautiful journey, friend, and a thoroughly rewarding experience that will help bring you more into your true, fulfilled powerful divine self.

Namaste. One Love, Jackie.

Table of Contents

Chapter One
Short History of Meditation
and Practice

"I think, therefore I am."
–René Descartes, French Philosopher, Mathematician and Scientist

According to my research online, and from reading the information shared on Wikipedia.org, it would appear that the Indian subcontinent is the first to depict the practice of sitting in a meditative state. Wall art dating back from 3,500 to 5,000 BCE depicts figures with eyes shut and legs crossed over. Various forms of meditation also developed in Taoist China and Buddhist Indian and Nepal around fifth/sixth centuries BCE.

However, I am sure this simple practice will have been much more ancient than this in my opinion with individuals including High priestesses, Druids, Medicine Women, Native American Indian Truth Keepers, Dream Weaver Aboriginals, Vedic and those from the Middle East. All these people would have communed with the living spirit within themselves and with animals, nature and etheric spirits besides the living consciousness of Mother/Father God or Great Spirit. I believe meditation would have begun when the first human began to contemplate survival and their place in the world.

Chapter Two
What Is the Rainbow Path
Meditation Series All About?

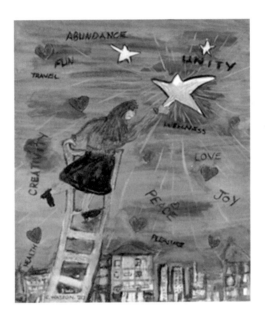

The Rainbow Path Meditation Series is a very loosely, semi-structured, gorgeous, spiritual and psychological development programme I began developing in 2004. This Series is created through incredible, visual, guided, inner-journeys that you will take.

Writing this meditation book is a new route for me to deliver a few of my one hundred and eighty odd Guided therapeutic meditations and spiritual adventures. I have previously been used to conducting my meditations in person and of late I have also moved online, with my beautiful evolving circles of amazing friends. (2020).

I feel confident that if you are in the right frame of mind, in a peaceful place that is dimmed, with no noise pollution or distractions, mobile or landline telephones switched to silent, then you should be able to gently regress into these meditations and come back out of them if you follow the same routine each and every time to begin a journey. The routine will be given just once to save repetition at the beginning of each meditation. Please do follow it diligently.

Obviously, you'll have to do the prep work—such as the breathwork that I will lead you through in the routine, next I hope you will be prepared and excited from reading the introduction that sets the mood and theme for what you will be about to experience in each meditation.

The other thing is you will have to have your eyes open to read and participate in the routine each time and also to read the storylines of each meditation but try your best to shut your eyes and tune in as often as you can, in order to get fully immersed in the journey and to really get the best out of each of them, psychically and on all levels. Tune in with your eyes closed for as long as it takes to connect and be in the zone; be in the visions.

There really are many benefits to be had in each of these beautifully crafted, most often channelled scripts/visions. There truly are many twists and turns, with hopefully some lights-on-moments of discovery too. These epiphanies you will experience may be subtle or profound. I have seen many of these moments occur for my Meditator companions and friends over the years of running my Circles, besides from my own personal experiences.

I developed 'The Rainbow Path Meditation Series' myself having attended a Circle whilst living in Adelaide, South Australia in 2004. I attended a Circle for one year and began to be inspired myself to write my own series of meditations. This Series is about being mindfully wide awake and increasing your sensitivities, or as I say your 'clairs', clairvoyance, clairaudience, claircognizant and general clair-knowingness.

You'll learn how to properly breathe, as most people on the planet shallow breathe. This is very much part of the repeated routine you'll undertake prior to going on a meditation journey.

Breathwork is so important to help you achieve that calm, quiet mind and body required to go into a semi-trance or meditative state.

Doing the routine you'll connect and strengthen the connection to The Creator, whether that be Mother or Father God or Great Spirit to you or just Universal energy. If you have not managed this connection in the past, I can promise it is a beautiful experience if you are a believer.

Hopefully, as you travel through these pages, you will connect into the essence and spirit of the Rainbow Path and all of us kindred spirits that have travelled these journeys before you, or indeed, right now, somewhere online or perhaps in a personal circle. Remember you are not alone. We acknowledge you right now. Tune in to us too. Our special essence and magic are right here on these pages.

We also link heart-to-heart and hand-in-hand around the Pillar of Light, this happens every time we connect personally or through online classes. The Pillar of light is where people we love and care for can be invited (telepathically) to receive love, support or healing if needed, in accordance with their divine will. It is part of the ceremony or wee ritual we do every single time we begin meditation. Many people have acknowledged the benefit they have experienced from this through letters or passing messages of thanks on to the Circles.

How Is Rainbow Path Meditation Series Structured?
The Routine to Follow

Refer back to this section and follow this routine every single time you wish to go on a meditation journey.

Settling Down and Breathwork

Get comfortable in your chair or bed. Take a deep breath, in through your mouth and out through your mouth, really connect to your breath as you place your hands on your lower abdomen. You want to bring the breath down into this whole region. It will oxygenate your body and at the same time help you get into a pace and rhythm that will aid you relaxing deeper and deeper.

Breathe in through your mouth and out through your mouth, in through your mouth and out through your mouth. Do some more and shut your eyes as often as you can to help you take your focus within. This also helps you block out distractions around you. Breathe again in through your mouth and out through your mouth into your lower abdomen. Deep rhythmic, yogic breaths. Do five of these now.

Feel your head, neck and shoulders begin to drop and relax and, then your chest and back. Take a couple of nice breaths in through your nose next for a count of five, exhaling out through your mouth. Feeling the stomach and abdomen, hips and whole pelvic girdle relax—feel yourself just melting into the chair, as if your head is also melting into your body like ice cream. All thoughts become less and less.

Soon you will feel all thoughts have dissipated completely. Your thighs, knees, calves and feet are softening and relaxing. How good it feels. Keep your eyes shut as often as you can after you have read and digested a chunk of information as you continue now and when you begin to go into a meditation, only opening them to read the script; as I said it helps you focus within and everything you are going to experience in this book will be inside you.

Connecting with Mother/Father God or Great Spirit

Now tilt your head upwards and with your eyes shut, use your inner vision to see and connect with the light of Creation, Great Spirit, Mother/Father God—whatever you may call this Light and loving consciousness. Sense an outpouring, down-pouring of beautiful pearlescent light, gently spilling down towards you through the cosmos, universe and galaxy into our galaxy and atmosphere. Sense your head tingling in response and the top of your crown opening up to receive this beautiful light. Smile in gratitude of this pure, loving light as it soaks and saturates over your whole aura and in through your mind and body.

Smile. Feel it. How good it feels. Feeling the connection to the rest of creation is good. Feel the light pouring down your legs and out the bottom of your feet, into the very core and heart of our beautiful planet. Imagine yourself as a vessel a conduit that is connecting the heavens with our beautiful pristine Earth. Send a puff of love down into the centre of the Earth and take a moment just to say thank you.

Thank you for the shelter, abundance, protection, nourishment and beauty we receive every day. Thank you. Now send a puff of love up to the Great Spirit, all love of creation, for the unseen subtle guidance we receive everyday keeping us on track. Give thanks for the Spirit that we are and that we are also part of the Creator or Great Spirit. Thank you.

Pillar of Light

Focus on the painting I have created for you of the Pillar of Light, Imagine that this translucent column of energy is full of iridescent, translucent, conscious loving energy from Source that anchors in the very heart of our Newly blossoming New World. One we create with our thoughts words and actions. If you are in a circle with others, then visualise a pillar of light with each participant connecting with one another around this shimmering column as it descends from the Cosmos, from the Great Spirit. Opalescent, quintessence light. Feel how vibrant, alive and conscious it really is and how much potent healing energy is pulsing up and down it. Beautiful.

Call in a loved one or anyone you wish to offer a helping hand to that is perhaps struggling in your mind to just step into the Pillar of Light now, for love support or healing. Remember, it must be in accordance with the loved one's own divine will to receive it. This is Universal/Cosmic Law. If someone wishes to have a life experience that involves an illness or pain and suffering then you are not permitted to interfere and affect their karma.

Each individual is going through their own experiences in life and we must always respect them even if we want to try and rescue them from suffering, if that person you call upon silently in your mind does not step forward and you don't see them in your third eye vision, then it means they do not want to join you and step into the healing Pillar of Light. It is their choice to go through their own challenge alone.

Light Body

Step out of your dense physical body now, which is a light-body—a mirror of yourself. I will guide you safely back at the very end of each of the meditation journeys and ground or earth you where you will feel anchored back safely. You will also be guided to do a technique to protect your energy field or aura with the assistance of Archangel Michael and His Legion of Foot Soldiers or Beams of Light if you prefer this image. It's safe to journey with me.

The Pillar of Light

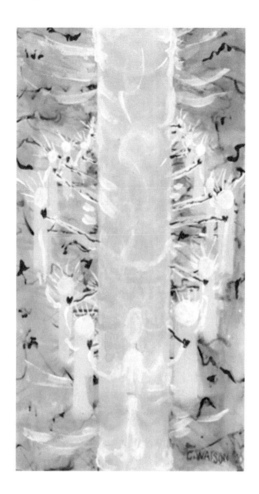

End of Routine

You'll discover, by the end of this book, and having completed each Meditation that you have more knowledge of the inner workings of yourself, you'll have made incredible new connections with your inner male and female self, your inner child, archangels and saints also aspects of Divine 'Great Mother Goddess'. The connections you make and the messages you receive may be strong, or perhaps subtle. However, they will all hopefully result in you feeling more supported and guided in your life.

It is a bit of a 'homecoming' journey, best enjoyed if you read this book with a touch of child-like wonder and an open heart, just as many people have before you. You will become part of the Rainbow Path's beautiful 'Soul-Tribe'—and you are most welcome, I can assure you.

You will learn about sacred rituals and ceremonies and history as I bring this into some of my scripts. I like to think of myself as an Educator. I often fancied becoming a Teacher when I was a wee young one, laying out questionnaires for my four siblings, being the eldest of my Tribe. I also had a very short stint of wanting to be a Nun, (I liked the long black tunic and white head veil/the habit they wore).

I will lead you as your personal Mentor and Guide to some very sacred sites and to experience the real essence of these places that will be imbued within your consciousness. All in all, it is a multi-dimensional, colourful, magical, informative, healing and individual experience you can expect from coming along with me for the ride. I hope you enjoy it. We've been expecting you, beautiful Soul!

Other Ways to Continue with this Rainbow Path Journey

If you have enjoyed and benefited from this Series of journeys, then know there are another hundred and seventy odd more of them. Yes, indeed! I have been guiding circles for nearly two decades. What is just amazing is you could be sitting in a jungle in the Amazon or the outback of Australia (as long as you have Wi-Fi and a laptop/smartphone), and join in with one of my Meditation circles online. You can Join the gorgeous family of meditators, from the comfort of your own home. How cool is that?

Email carolwatson_au@yahoo.com in the first instance and get in touch, from there we can exchange mobile numbers to arrange either a 'WhatsApp' or 'Zoom' class.

Chapter Three
Benefits of Mindfulness Meditation

There is real scientific research now on the benefits of mindful meditation that a lot of Meditation Teachers, like myself, are thrilled about, having waited an awfully long time for it to come to the fore. Here is the awareness that I have gathered from my twenty years of meditating. Alongside each note I have included my thoughts on the benefits, to make it easy to glance through.

1. Mindfulness Meditation helps filter through our thoughts, as we begin to learn how to take back our self-control from those persistent, negative ones.
2. Thousands of thoughts are repeated every hour of every day and the majority are negative. It creates a downward spiral for us.
3. Meditation allows us to clear the clutter in our heads, which then gives us space for new and more empowering thoughts to enter that are more life-enhancing.
4. Research shows that Meditation brings divergent thinking. This type of thinking allows for new wonderful ideas to be generated. Our creativity is activated. In just eleven hours, that is all it takes for the structural change in our brains to happen when we meditate.
5. Meditation can extend your life span by up to ten years.
6. Meditation helps us focus and have deeper self-control.
7. It releases stress and tension.
8. Meditation can bring us into a state of deep peace, even euphoria.
9. Things are put back into perspective when we meditate.
10. We reclaim the inner territory we perhaps may have let go off or suppressed within us. This allows us to not only face our inner fears and phobias but to begin the process of healing them.

11. We become more self-empowered.

12. The relationship with the self improves exponentially and also strengthens the relationships with other people in your life.

13. Meditation is therapeutic and healing.

14. You can connect better with your breath and breathing pattern.

15. By breathing better and more deeply in a rhythmic fashion you release carbon dioxide and take in life-enhancing oxygen. This is therapeutic and healing.

16. You connect much more with your inner and external world and with other people.

17. The connection to the Galaxy, Universe and to the Great Spirit is increased.

18. The connection and appreciation to all life is increased.

19. Through meditation, your empathy, compassion, appreciation, gratitude and love increases enormously. Your heart is more open and receptive.

20. Through meditation, you touch into your Soul and make a lasting and loving acquaintance.

21. Through guided meditation and visualisations, you will get to experience magical, sensory, exquisite visions. These will be both uplifting and life-enhancing.

22. Psychic art and self-expression will increase.

23. Through guided meditations on the chakra system you will be able to see and clear dense areas. The meditations will equip you with the ability to clear these areas and feel rejuvenated.

24. Your confidence will increase.

25. You will be able to see the bigger picture in life with greater clarity.

26. You will become less egotistical and more expansive.

27. By going on guided journeys, you will learn how to manifest the life you want and gain the spiritual and psychological tools to steer you on the right path.

28. You will learn how to connect on a deep level with the animal and plant kingdoms.

29. An appreciation for nature is born.

30. A deep sense of peace and well-being will happen, and continuous meditation will ensure this feeling is sustained. It becomes sustained.

31. You will learn how to sculpt your own life as you see fit.

32. Through the 'Rainbow Path Meditation Series' you will learn how to sense elements and other life forms, such as spirit, Archangels and, deceased loved ones etc.

33. You will lose the fear of death because you will come to understand life is perpetual.

34. You will begin to stop thinking about, "how can I best serve 'ME'?" and will instead consider "how can I best serve the world?"

35. Life just gets better, richer, fuller, happier and with much more meaning when meditation becomes a part of life.

36. Meditation helps you realise just how great it is to be alive and teaches you to value every moment.

Chapter Four
Feedback from Regular
Rainbow Path Meditators

March – July 2020: Global Quarantine

I have run Guided Meditation Circles for many years from my home, from Clinics, Yoga Studios, Cafes etc and always in person. However, during the time of the global COVID-19 pandemic, I began offering and running many weekly online meditation classes from my home. The move online was due to the closure of the clinic and Yoga studios that I usually worked from as, similar to many businesses, there were concerns regarding newly imposed safety guidelines and the virus.

I must confess; I am not a techno-geek—more the opposite! So it delighted me to challenge myself to start the new venture of setting up small, intimate 'WhatsApp' video calls, and running hourly meditation circles online. (See, we always learn, even when things are challenging or difficult. In fact, usually when things are challenging or difficult…right?) It helps us face our fears and often, somehow, enables us to stretch deeper and further, into a more resourceful and happy self. Agreed?

On that note, these are the creative expressions and feedback that some of my beautiful inspired meditation companions shared with me, describing their journey with me during this testing but reflective time.

Jeannie Thompson, Essex, England, UK

"During the lockdown, I was moored on a twenty-eight-foot boat with limited resources to entertain myself. I ended up then in a three-foot tent when the boat needed to be moored for repair work. Carol's Rainbow Path Meditation Series (guided online), helped me on so many levels during these

challenging times—community, laughter, adventure, magic, guides, colour and healing. A beautiful space holder, she is that I am forever grateful for."

Jacqueline Evenes, Edinburgh, Scotland

Jacqueline has been in one of my longest-running meditation circles, coming in and out of it over the past decade and a half. She has always supported my work and has loved the connection with everyone, besides the learning and growth she has often told me she has gained from it. As she once told me the Rainbow Path Meditation Series of spiritual teachings truly was a foundation for the course her spiritual life journey took. I have always felt humbled and delighted to have Jacqueline with her own lovely wisdom on board.

"The Jack in the Beanstalk/World Tree meditation, meeting the ancient Fortingal Yew Tree and descending into the underworld, through an Oak tree, to meet my power animal on the loch, inspired me. I experienced the 'All' of the 'Tree', all power, 'root-soul' connection and the rooting network of connection with the Rainbow Path Meditation Circle."

Bridie Docherty, Edinburgh, Scotland

"Rainbow Path Meditation Series—the online circle has helped keep me grounded and calm. I have been a regular with Carol for over a year now too. It is a very supportive group and I have made wonderful connections with like-minded people."

Jasmine Birch, Edinburgh, Scotland

Jasmine has been a regular over the past fifteen years with the Rainbow Path Meditation Series, dipping in and out where time allows especially during the months of 'lock-down' enforced upon everyone country-wide. Here she gives it in her words.

"Creating from our journey together—letting go—letting flow—opening to unconditional light and love. A single divine journey within a divine four—within the greater Rainbow Path circle. Within all circles, we journey within the circle of life. Blessings—gratitude and divine transformation for myself and

all... 'Om Shanti Om'. I am a being of Violet Fire, I am the purity of God's desire."

Lily Gardener

"I had been attending Carol's meditation classes for more years than I can really remember. It had a very special, magical, quality and was an incredibly supportive, non-judgemental space. These classes were a reflection of Carol's essence and of the individuals in the Circles. The Rainbow Path Tribe was a wonderful group of people, individually and as a unit for me. I am so grateful to have been part of it over the years. I always sensed the support from the Circles as being very nourishing and loving and won't ever forget that."

Kareen McQueen, Edinburgh, Scotland

"To feel your heart, to unite with your soul, to realise our inter-relatedness with the Universe and our sacred Mother Earth. The Rainbow Path Meditations have enhanced my personal journey in a loving and relaxed way. What's not to love!"

Rumi Lipinski, USA

"The experiences of the Rainbow Path Meditation Series for me, I would like to watching a movie and enjoying it even more, as it has felt almost like immersive entertainment, and definitely better for the soul. I have been able to transport myself to a different world, thanks to Carol."

Joslin Lambert, Edinburgh, Scotland

"Love the meditations in the Rainbow Path Series. They are very calming and reflective. I have experienced a range of vibrant colours during meditation while also feeling more connected to the natural world. I will be continuing with these online classes into the future."

Felicity Clyne, Edinburgh, Scotland

"My mandala-like tree/nature artworks reflect the nature journey's we have been guided on in the Rainbow Path Meditation Series: Jack and The Beanstalk/World Tree, Fortingal Yew Tree. The Gardener etc. My pictures are

quite abstract, however, they represent a door to the other realm, the other world."

Samantha Thomson, Edinburgh, Scotland

"I find the Rainbow Path Meditation Circle gatherings very enlightening. A place of wonder and self-discovery."

Maureen Skylark, Edinburgh, Scotland

"I was attending Carol Watson's Rainbow Path Meditation Series of Meditations in one of her Circle's online, during the COVID-19 Pandemic in 2020, and I found it to be such an uplifting, calming and peaceful experience.

"Carol has a soothing meditative voice that really impacted on lessening my stress levels, having suffered from complex trauma since childhood.

"I so enjoyed the wonderful visionary journeys she led us on, as they acted as a catalyst for opening up my imagination and helping me to experience my own fabulous visionary world. The delightful journeys were a joy and so vividly described that I had found deeper meaning and peace from them.

"Carol always begins with the breathwork and then brings in the ebullient light-filled cosmic/universal/galactic energy, (The Pillar of Light), primarily through the crown of your head and down through the body. This helps to cleanse anything negative. I did find it empowering to take time to focus on healing my body.

"Each meditation was beautifully described and usually led to a sacred place, often culminating at a temple or zenith or pool. This often felt transcendent and even celestial at times.

"What is extraordinary, is that as a group we were able to share our journey's, which may for some feel totally over one's normal sphere of thought, however, it's an escape from the mundane and the real issues of the modern world.

"On a personal, spiritual level, the meditations helped me connect with the Great Universal consciousness and I tried to take what wisdom I could from any messages from the symbolism of the meditations. What was incredible was that the group members usually found some commonality within the group experiences, whether that was with the healing colours we experienced, crystals or vision.

"Life is a journey, and it's good to acknowledge that dreams and our visionary world are part of us and that we can gain wisdom from our own subconscious minds."

Elaine Katherine McLean, Edinburgh, Scotland

"Rainbow Path Meditations totally destress me and clears my head of all the rubbish that is attached to my pain, I suffer daily. It puts me into a happy, happy place."

Heather Erskine, Edinburgh, Scotland

"I moved to an area in Edinburgh Carol Watson was running her beautiful Meditation Circles from. I have enjoyed every one of them …. Carol lead me onto her 'Rainbow Path' and I became one of the 'Rainbow Tribe' and I love it.

"Carol has taken us on some amazing, mysterious journeys by listening to her tell you the story. I've loved them all and they have helped me so much to have a positive frame of mind and to be able to find that magic place that you need to escape to at times. During the Pandemic of 2020, Carol encouraged us in the circles she runs to get involved in the creative project. She suggested we all do some sort of creative work that would reflect either a beautiful meditation she guided us through, or what we feel we have gained from the guided journey's, or on a personal level, to share self-reflective things that we each worked through.

"As an artist, I loved the Jack and The Beanstalk tree meditation, it has been my favourite to date, with the amazing tree house and did my best to reflect this in my paintings. It stretched me creatively to try new subjects I would not have attempted before, and I thoroughly enjoyed it.

"I felt the power of the beam of light, in her 'Pillar of Light' painting and I love the imagery of all of us holding hands around it and heart-to-heart connecting, which we do each and every time we get together whether in person or online.

"I have loved every one of the meditations and felt so supported during this pandemic time of 2020. I have felt so grateful to be part of the Rainbow Path Meditation Tribe. I look forward to many more journeys ahead. How exciting!

"Thank you, Carol, you are an amazing storyteller and an amazing lady. Thank you for inviting me into your magic."

The poems that are about to follow are written by two participants from my meditation circle, who have kindly allowed me to share their poems; the inspiration for which they have gathered from my guided meditations.

The Tree House Poem
Heather Erskine

I climb up a tree, I feel I can breathe. I feel I can see everything.
The nature, the magic up in the sky. I feel like I can fly.
I go inside to the cosy tree house. I feel so cosy, as snug as a bug in a rug.
Like a wee mouse, cosy in my tree house.
I listen to the birds as they sing, the sunshine pouring in.
This magical tree house, I could stay here forever; read a book, drink some tea, chat to the birds and nature…….. that will do for me!

2020 Vision
Jeannie Thompson

Once upon a time, the world closed down. Not a sound could be heard, even from this tiny town.

Owl sat on his branch and basked in the peace. Rotating his head, he hooted to the geese.

They honked their salute and swan upstream. The story, my friend, is not as it would seem.

On this water, there also lived a boat. Inside you would find a witch and pet stoat.

Scratching her head, she admitted defeat. Too much free time. 'Is it ok to go eat?'

The stoat shook his head, in utter disgust. 'Stop overeating or you'll simply go burst.'

An owl flew past and circled overhead. 'What does he whisper instead of going to bed?'

Jeanne sought magic, whispers and dreams. Living on the edge of the otherworld team.

An argument kicked off upon the bow. Three cranes had landed and started a row.

'What are you doing?'

'What is all this noise?'

'We bring a reminder of the wonder of your voice.'

'I don't understand, what can you mean?'

'The answer my friend is asking you be seen.'

Jeannie rolled her eyes. She didn't know why but being around people often made her sigh.

Tripping over a goblet, the water started to spill. 'A leak in your essence is a gap in your skills.'

'Look all around you, not a moment to lose. Nature is a community that leaves us clues.'

'Boredom is the mark of a missing soul-part. Use the time wisely to make a new start.'

'Look deep into the watery abyss. What can you see? What is amiss?'

Squirrel popped aboard and scuttled up the mast. 'Look up ahead. The ocean is vast.'

Bat was there, sitting on the crow's nest. Wearing a smile and a yellow string vest.

A hawk appeared and joined the crew. A party it seemed, would only take a few.

Sitting by the helm, Jeannie found a key. The most beautiful flower she ever did see.

Hawk Mother, she smiled, as she held out her wing.

'Your inner beauty, my friend, has asked to sing.'

Treasure awaits all those that are brave. The challenge you see is entering the cave.

We shall leave this story as quickly as it appeared.

But remember—remember—unleash your inner weird.

Your heart it calls, a story, re-write.

The hero will journey and your soul will ignite.

The end for now, but all shall be revealed. Nature is calling and dreaming a new deal.

Blessings to your path. May you dance and may you laugh.

Chapter Five
Power of Affirmations

What is an 'affirmation' and how can I implement them into my life to enhance it?

As it says, it's an affirmative statement, sentence or even a word that can uplift, motivate, or move you energetically, emotionally, mentally or spiritually—or indeed all of the fore-mentioned.

To understand the real benefits of the positive power that words and statements have, it's important to take a moment to 'feel into' the negative ones first. Don't worry, we'll only take a minute here and move through it into the light of power-words. However, it is important to experience the difference so you can properly appreciate the power held by words. Experience is everything, right?

Call up the word 'fear' in your mind when you think of something that is frightening that you still wrestle with; a phobia, being abandoned or something else awful. Feel it and contemplate how constricting it is. Anger; feel its energy, it tightens everything up like a knot inside as does rage and hatred. These words are very powerful indeed, and you know the impact it has on you when you experience these moments of deep negativity.

You are debilitated, frozen, lifeless even. You shrink and feel shrivelled. You feel awful and loathe yourself. Just see how it spirals ever downward. It can reach such a low place that people need medication and that doesn't always resolve everything. Often, it just puts a sticky plaster or Band-Aid on a seeping puss spot. You shrink, you withdraw, you isolate yourself—you wither.

OK, let's get into the light side of things. Contrary to negative words, words of positive affirmation have a profound positive impact on our mental state. Add positive affirmations in a sentence or statement and look how potent and alive the message is. When we give a repeated positive message to ourselves over a twenty-one day period or longer, the mind is unable to distinguish between fact and fiction.

These are the first steps towards the end goal of manifestation. Know that you need to think something, say it out loud, repeat it to the Universe and then physically take steps to put the plan into action. Thinking alone does nothing. I can assure you of this fact as I did years of affirmations without putting anything into practice and nothing came of them. Live the life you desire through your thoughts, words and actions—that's the motto for success.

Some Incredibly Powerful Affirmations to Work With

1. I am abundant in every way.
2. I love myself, I am loving and loved. I am blessed.
3. I am perfect in all my imperfections as is everyone else.
4. I discern everything but am moving to accept everything just the way they are.
5. We are all one.
6. I am grateful for everything in my life.
7. I am enough!
8. I connect with nature and all living things and see wonder through my eyes.
9. You are perfect, I am perfect.
10. I manifest the life I choose.
11. I am the architect of my world.
12. I am so grateful to all the people in my life that care, share and love me.
13. I am supported. I support others.
14. Empathy and compassion flow through me.
15. I am creative and alive and so grateful.
16. I magnetise the right situations to me.
17. I am growing and learning all the time.
18. I am connected and tuned in to Source who gently guides my journey.
19. I honour my ancestors and remember them all.
20. I respect myself and others.
21. What good deeds I do today will come back to me. It is the law of karma.

22. I don't give to receive. I give with an open heart.
23. I am full of child-like wonder, awe and magic.
24. I know how to let my hair down and play.
25. I am tuned into the wisdom of Sophia. Great Mother Goddess.
26. Everything is in complete and perfect balance within me.
27. I listen to my heart.
28. I am in tune with my beautiful soul.
29. You are me, I am you. We are all one.
30. I know peace and live a peaceful, harmonious life with dignity and respect for all.

Chapter Six
Relaxed, Mindful Presence

Make yourself comfortable in your chair or bed. Start to breathe in through your open mouth and out through your mouth in deep, rhythmic breaths, known as yogic breathing. Place your hands on your lower abdomen and take the depth of your breath right down and into this region, oxygenating those organs and the whole intestinal region.

Guide your big breath deep; draw it in and down through your mouth, into your chest and lungs and down into your stomach. Feel the abdomen expand, feel it. Now go deeper into your whole abdomen and deep down into the lower abdomen and pelvis. Feel the breath filling your whole body with this beautiful oxygen. Continue to breathe really deep, long breaths, in through your mouth and out through your mouth.

As you breathe, you will notice you are fully focused solely on the act of breathing, and not any thoughts. Think about how good this feels. It is easy and effortless to breathe deep and exhale all the toxins and carbon dioxide out.

Focus on how you feel centred and still at the moment, completely present, right now. Keep focusing on your breath. It feels great, doesn't it? Nothing else matters, just breathing in and out. It's empowering, right?

Now focus on relaxing the breath, to gentler, softer breaths. It's so wonderful and easy to breathe.

Feel yourself mindful of your position, the seat you are in, how comfortable or uncomfortable you feel. Wriggle to get as settled and comfortable as you possibly can.

Feel the mind quieten, with less chit chat, less activity and how good that feels too. Give a nice deep sigh. Ahhhh. This is the sound of the heart. Ahhhhh.

Feel aware and mindful of how your shoulders are as you allow them to soften and relax. Breathe out.

Feel the whole chest cavity and lungs relax. Sigh; ahhhhh.

Notice how your stomach and abdomen feel; is there any tension here? If so, breathe into it to soften it.

Feel the whole hip girdle and the pelvis relax, sink or melt into the chair. How good it feels to be body-conscious, mindful of your whole mind, body and feelings. How good is it to be self-aware? Very, very good yes?

Taking the time out to simply sit at peace, be present and still and relaxed is amazing, right? Feel the heaviness in your thighs and calves relax, and then in the feet. Feel them lighter and softer, easier. Feel a flow through the whole mind and body as you take your focus up to your head and sense light pouring in through it. Notice how it soothes you, connecting you to the Great Spirit, to the light of Creation, and how wonderfully connected you feel right now in this moment.

Breathe once again deeper, this time in through your nose and out through your mouth. Place your tongue on the roof of your mouth now, as you breathe in through your nose and out through your mouth. Suck the oxygen in nice and deep and focus it filling your throat, mouth, cheeks, face, your whole head, your whole mind. Do another five of these very powerful breaths. Now go back to breathing normally, making it more shallow.

You may feel slightly lightheaded—this is due to the surge of oxygen, it will settle in you soon.

Sense a gentle light flowing from the atmosphere and galaxy, a beautiful influx of light. Know that you are connecting to the universal abundance of love and light as it pours down and over you; running through you head to toe. How well it feels, knowing you are part of everything; An inter-connected Consciousness. How good does it feel as you feel a flow and a warm glow throughout your whole body head to toe? Contemplate your feet and how they feel on the floor, feeling grounded and connected to the Earth.

Allow this beautiful light to pour through your body from your head, right down to your feet and out the bottom of your soles into the earth beneath you. Feel roots anchoring you to the new earth you are creating with your thoughts, words and actions. Feel grounded.

Feel a light all around you like a buoyant cushion of extra support and protection. Know you can ask for this anytime during the day or week ahead and work with it. Practice this 'mindfulness presence' meditation to get you fully aligned anytime you feel out of whack or low—or when you're anxious or perhaps just tired with all your thoughts flooding in.

How good has this exercise been and useful to you? Pat your thighs and wiggle your toes, taking a deep breath, while lifting and dropping your shoulders. Bring yourself back into your room and space, smile at how good things are in the moment. Nothing else matters just how you feel right here and right now. Nothing else matters. Smile. Now open your eyes and smile. Feel revived and re-energised!

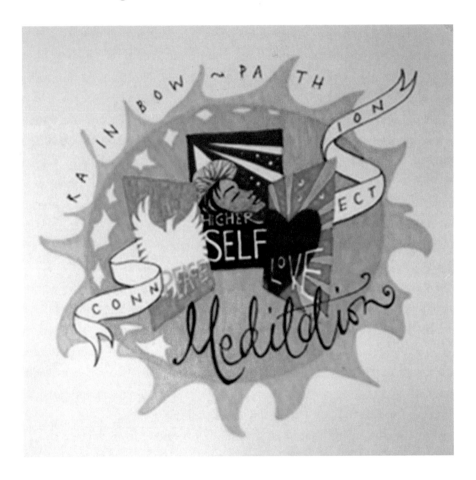

Artwork by Samantha Thomson

Chapter Seven
Rainbow Ribbons

A colour healing journey to discover what colour (s) you are needing replenished with.

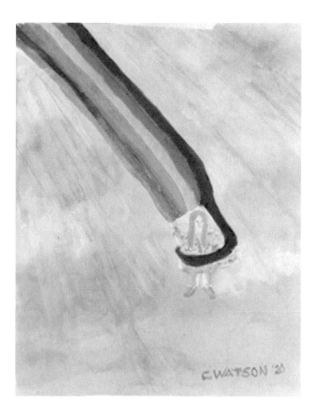

C.WATSON '20

[Begin the routine. Refer to Chapter Two.]

As you step out of your dense body and into your light body, you step into a glorious meadow with long green grass, speckled with buttercups and daisies. Can you see them? The sun is shining and the clouds are so white and fluffy in a turquoise sky. Smell the aromas, feel the ground beneath your feet, sense the warm air blowing all around you and through your hair, kissing your cheeks. What an incredible, happy, glorious day this is. Feel it.

Speak for a moment inside you, ask what colours are depleted in your energy field, chakras. Ask the colour (or colours) you most need to respond to your request. They will show themselves as one or more from the rainbow ribbons that begin to form way up in the sky. Look up, see them. Streams of heavenly rainbow colours dancing and twisting and blowing in the wind. Can you see them?

How incredible they look, right? They begin to descend and sway on the breeze look at them all, the poppy red, the ocean blue, the violet, the sunshine yellow, what other colours do you see? What colour or colours are calling to you, reaching into your heart and soul. Watch them flow and twirl in the breeze as they descend towards you now. See them.

How does it make you feel? What a blessed day this truly is. These are heavenly iridescent rainbow rays you are seeing. Is it a cooling colour you see coming to you now, or a warm colour or colours? They coil around you and lift you up now; as if you are as light as a feather. Feel it. You are off the ground and weightless. How fantastic this feels, right?

NB. Orange oil is for stimulating the abdomen or core, and energy booster oil; ideal if it is the red or orange ribbons and chakras. Woodland oil is good for the green chakra, earthy heart-opening energy. Peppermint oil is cool and calming and helps with any inflammation, and is a great oil to connect with the blue or the throat chakra or body in general. Citrine essence is for the yellow ray.

Feel absorbed in the oil essence and the colour ray(s), as you see way up ahead in the sky a double-arched rainbow—see it. Feel your heart open and expand and allow your Inner Child to rise in you to join you as you go to the very arch of the highest rainbow. How amazing this feels. You are going to slide down it like a shoot.

You are in the arms of your colour rays too, remember, but the colours of the rainbow will absorb deeper into you—all the spectrum of the rainbow as you slide down this shoot for a while. Try it now and enjoy as you whizz and squeal down the slide. How exciting and invigorating. Do it again, and again. It's your time, your journey—so go enjoy. One final go; head to the very top, the arch of the rainbow.

The other rainbow energy seems to saturate into this first stronger one, and a deep encased tube is created. Feel encapsulated fully in it, like a flume at the swimming pool. Push off and slide down it, feeling the depth of the rainbow inside every muscle of your body; every organ, your bones and cells. This is amazing, right? Do it once more and then the rainbow ribbons you are coiled in will come away and take you down to the ground and back to your physical self. Make it count, last go. Enjoy.

As you exit the end of the tunnel (or flume), the rainbow rays you are surrounded in breeze away from the rainbows and swirl you through the air, gently twisting this way and that way. It is such a beautiful sensation, right? Feel the fizz and sparkle in your body and in your cells. Say your thank you now to the oils and colour rays as you descend to the ground and are dropped upright on your feet; back in front of your physical you.

Bringing Yourself Back into Your Physical Body

It's time to return. See the physical you, standing there, arms wide open welcoming you back with a big smile. Walk towards your physical self and go around the back of you. Step into your physical body one leg at a time, like a hand slipping back into a glove. One arm, then your other arm. Bring your torso back into the body and head.

Instantly you are transported back into your room and chair. Feel the weight on your shoulders and your feet grounding you. Sense your spirit fully back and present in your body. Take some really deep breaths again; in through your mouth and out through your mouth into the lower abdomen. Now take two or three in through your nose and out through your mouth. Feel yourself in your chair now.

Grounding/Anchoring Yourself and Golden Bubble of Protection

Sense golden roots coming out of your feet and grounding you on the most beautiful earth. Feel it. Sense a golden bubble all around your aura; it is like extra skin—a layer of protection. It is strong and pliable but impenetrable. Feel it. This golden bubble will be activated indefinitely to protect your energy from negative people or anything environmental. Smile. Take a moment just to say thank you to your body. Your heart, your mind, your soul. Finally, open your eyes whenever you feel ready.

Review

Feel renewed; feel at peace, present and joyful. Take notes in your diary—you can read back and reflect on it all when you need to. If you are meditating in a group then allow each person the opportunity to share what magic they have experienced, remembering all the good moments.

What did you feel, see, sense, or just know? What lessons can you take away from this that will help you in any way with your beautiful life journey? What colour or colours wrapped you up in their ray and how did the colour (s) affect you in your body? Read up on the Chakra system to learn what particular colour can do to influence your whole system. Perhaps this area was or is slightly depleted and needs restoring to its full glory. Eating colours or wearing colours helps you absorb that spectrum into the body and co-assist your energy levels there. Smile.

Chapter Eight
Jack and the Beanstalk

How can you rise, friend, if you don't mobilise and stretch upwards within and out-with yourself!

"You must be the change you wish to see in the world!"

– Gandhi

Settling Down and Breathwork

Then follow the full routine before going on your journey.

Get comfortable in your chair. Take a deep breath and let it out; now shut your eyes and breathe, in through your mouth and out through your mouth into your lower abdomen. Deep rhythmic, yogic breaths. Do five of these now. Feel your head, neck and shoulders begin to drop and relax and, then your chest and back.

Take a couple of nice breaths in through your nose next to five exhaling out through your mouth. Feeling the stomach and abdomen, hips and whole pelvic girdle relax—feel yourself just melting into the chair. Your thighs, knees, calves and feet are softening and relaxing. How good it feels.

Keep your eyes shut throughout the whole guided meditation, only opening them to read the script; it helps you focus within. It's safe to journey with me. Come, join me on this magical, mystical, fun adventure. Bring out your inner child-self and let's have some fun.

Visualise yourself walking into an old wood; smell its musk and feel the mischievousness of this secret forest. Shortly, you are going to meet with a magical huge tree. You will also meet the fairy or elementals that reside in or around the tree. On you go—explore, skip, sing, dance, as you head for the interior of the woods. As you look at the tree canopy above and around you,

you spot one huge tree sticking out the top and into the clouds. You see it is the beanstalk tree. Head for it.

You see it come into view and pause to take in the ginormous size of its girth, and the canopy of leaves that surround it. You see thick branch-like limbs all the way up it, and what appears to be a tiny tree house in the clouds wrapped around the whole tree. Ask the tree if you can bless it with your sacred elixir, your magical new earth potion and if you can also climb it. On you go, ask. Smile as you say thank you for the privilege as the beanstalk welcomes you to do so.

On you go. Encircle the tree, running your hand round its base. Bless it with your spray. Now when you are ready, look for the foot and handholds that run all the way up the tree—this is going to be a mighty climb. In fact, it will be the climb of your life. Breathe and get mentally prepared. When you are ready step up onto the beanstalk and find your grip, look up for the next hold and so forth as you go, getting into a nice rhythm. How good does this feel?

Call out to the fairies or elemental beings to come and meet you as you climb. What do you feel and see?

Give your thanks as you continue your ascent into the heavens, through the tree canopy. The air feels different; you feel more free, there is not so much inner chatter. It's as if things have generally quietened down from the world you live in too. You feel a sense of disconnection from the busy world and people. It feels good.

As you rise you begin to look below and see a different perspective. You are near the heavens, immersed in clouds. Pause to consider what this beanstalk tree can help you understand about life and perspectives, your own viewpoints? Things really look so different when you look at things below from a great height. You see a broader, wider picture. What can you take away from this and use or integrate in your daily life?

Up above you, you see the tree house structure; climb up to it and go get yourself settled in there. You find cushions, a notebook and a blanket are there for you to rest and journal. Enjoy. In the tree house, you feel like you are almost in-between dimensions and worlds. A foot in heaven and a foot on Earth. How does that feel?

Is there anyone from the spirit world that wants to connect with your right now? This is your time, it's perfectly safe to do so. Just enjoy the quiet connection.

What and who did you see or sense? What message do they bring you? Always give your grateful thanks. After they have disappeared, it's time you leave the tree house and descend back into your realm. Find your foothold and head down. If you feel you would love to launch as a bird then do so and fly down the beanstalk instead—it's up to you. Feel the air change as you descend, feel the energy change.

Make sure to remember all your encounters so you can ponder on them after this journey has ended, and reflect in your own journal at home. Having a personal diary or journal is so therapeutic and useful. You can write about the visions and feelings you experienced and how it all made you feel. When you feel gloomy you can open and read the exciting information you gained from gorgeous trips like this one. Remember that you have experienced pure magic and you have truly been very blessed. Smile. As you reach and leap off the bottom of the beanstalk tree you see yourself. The physical you.

Bringing Yourself Back into Your Physical Body

It's time to return. See the physical you, standing there, arms wide open welcoming you back with a big smile. Walk towards your physical self and go around the back of you. Step into your physical body one leg at a time, like a hand slipping back into a glove. One arm, then your other arm. Bring your torso back into the body and head.

Instantly you are transported back into your room and chair. Feel the weight on your shoulders and your feet grounding you. Sense your spirit fully back and present in your body. Take some really deep breaths again; in through your mouth and out through your mouth into the lower abdomen. Now take two or three in through your nose and out through your mouth. Feel yourself in your chair now.

Grounding/Anchoring Yourself and Golden Bubble of Protection

Sense golden roots coming out of your feet and grounding you on the most beautiful earth. Feel it. Sense a golden bubble all around your aura; it is like extra skin—a layer of protection. It is strong and pliable but impenetrable. Feel it. This golden bubble will be activated indefinitely to protect your energy from negative people or anything environmental. Smile. Take a moment just to say

thank you to your body. Your heart, your mind, your soul. Finally, open your eyes whenever you feel ready.

Review

Feel renewed; feel at peace, present and joyful. Take notes in your diary— you can read back and reflect on it all when you need to. If you are meditating in a group then allow each person the opportunity to share what magic they have experienced, remembering all the good moments. What did you feel, see, sense, or just know? What lessons can you take away from this that will help you in any way with your beautiful life journey? Feel touched and blessed. Smile.

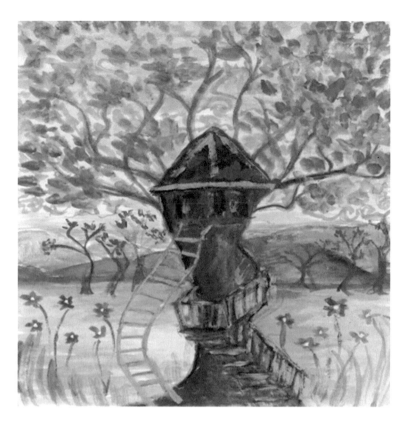

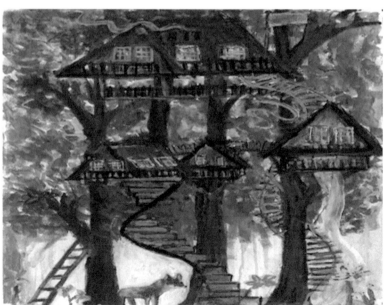

Artwork by Ele Elba

Chapter Nine
Healing Your Shadow

"It is our light and not our darkness that scares us so much."
– Nelson Mandela

"He who fears he will suffer, already suffers because he fears."
– Michel De Montaigne

We all have a light side that we love and like to portray to the world. However, each and every one of us has a dark side too, and it often can be the driver of our lives if we allow it to rule and control us. This meditation is hugely important in acknowledging aspects of this dark part of our make-up—our ego, our, shadow and our ancient reptilian part of our brain. The part that does the death roll and swallows us up (or anyone that truly threatens us in one gobble). We are not here to destroy our Shadow-Nature but to resolve the negative parts and integrate these aspects of us, fully healed into the 'LIGHT'.

According to some accounts, there are beings that are known as 'The Daughters of Darkness' that are around and can work with us if you feel you would like to explore this concept.

(Disclaimer/Footnote: Friend, It is my advice that if you are mentally not able to face your personal traumas or character challenging issues and feel this may be too much for you at this time, I strongly suggest you skip this mediation and move on the next one. If you need support with any negative struggles from your past perhaps, then do consider consulting an expert who can gently and professionally guide you through. Return to this meditation when you feel better equipped for it.)

Let's begin.

[Refer to your routine from Chapter Two first.]

Imagine you have entered into a darkened sanctuary. A quiet space. It feels safe and warm and comfortable.

Call upon your family and ancestors to integrate within us and ask all aspects of our Soul to come home to us (it has been known that the soul consists of one hundred and forty-four parts). Ask the Divine Mother Aspect of Source the Morrigan, to receive you into her incredible, deep, womb-like cave just a few steps in front. Do not allow yourself to halter or go into fear. There is nothing to fear bar fear itself.

Ask if you can meet the Great Mother of Darkness, The Morrigan. Sense this powerful energy source coming from the depth of the black void of the cave—towards the entrance and to you. What do you feel and what do you see? You now feel a strong sense of Her Presence very close and view her hand reaching out from the blackness to take hold of yours. She leads you gently into her cavern. Can you feel her? On you go, it is safe. It is a comforting feeling.

Conquer your fear and surrender to this moment as you take a step forward and enter a different vibration altogether, as you are immersed in the energy of the cave and Mother. Feel it.

Feel the living consciousness of this essence as you go deeper into the quiet blackness with Mother. How is it for you? Do you feel the power of the silence envelope you, soaking into your pores? How does this silence and darkness make you feel?

You are now led to the inner hub; the core of the cave where you see seated shadowy figures in a circle around a smouldering fire pit. The scene looks interesting and draws you towards it, even if you feel a little trepidation. You see there is a seat besides these Daughters of Darkness. Go and take a seat, as Mother leaves you to let you focus on the work you have to do.

These Guardians of Darkness absorb your fears when you choose to release them. liberating you from the chains of anxiety, stress, worry, negativity, phobias, limiting beliefs and fears. This is your time to sit with them and connect with them. Ask what they can show you in the black mirror on the floor near you. As you look into the mirror, it will come alive with images.

Ask the Guardians to show you your deepest darkness, your deepest fears. Allow whatever shows itself to rise from the reflections; feel it now rise inside you like a dormant lava lake. Do not be afraid, it is rising to be released. The energy of blackness will seep from you, as you let it go fully and wholly.

The energy will now absorb into the Daughters of Darkness. They love you and humanity so much and can help us let go of trauma and karma. They help us let go of repeated old, out-worn negative patterns. This is your time, make it count and enjoy the process.

Who have you spoken ill of and feel guilty about? What ill turn did you do to another that you have buried and tried to forget? Allow all of it to come up and rise within you, in order for it to then be released and leave you clear. Remember you can do this meditation as often as you need to fully purify your mind and body.

Feel a refreshing fizz in you or a cooling sensation as your cells, muscles, bones, organs get release. Feel it. How good does it feel to just acknowledge our burdens and hidden blackness? It is wonderful, right? There is so much more space in your mind for light and positive thoughts now. Space has been created and it feels good. Agreed?

Now it is time to give your deep thanks to each of these sacred Morrigan Priestesses. Go around the fire circle and bow to them. Take out the New Earth holy water and ask if you can bless them all individually, and give them each a pink rose quartz love heart stone.

You sense The Morrigan Mother coming forward now and the nurturing love you feel is overwhelming as she embraces you with the warmest heart hug you have ever had in your life. It is so stilling, soothing, calming and alive. Feel her heartbeat and feel your own begin to beat in tune with hers. She has an arm around your waist now as she walks you to the cave entrance. It is time to come back.

At the entrance, she hands you something. A keepsake gift. Take it and give your thanks. Hand your holy water new earth spray to her as a gift in return. Say your thank you, then bow and walk out of the cave, feeling ten times lighter than you entered.

Bringing Yourself Back into Your Physical Body

It's time to return. See the physical you, standing there, arms wide open welcoming you back with a big smile. Walk towards your physical self and go around the back of you. Step into your physical body one leg at a time, like a hand slipping back into a glove. One arm, then your other arm. Bring your torso back into the body and head.

Instantly you are transported back into your room and chair. Feel the weight on your shoulders and your feet grounding you. Sense your spirit fully back and present in your body. Take some really deep breaths again; in through your mouth and out through your mouth into the lower abdomen. Now take two or three in through your nose and out through your mouth. Feel yourself in your chair now.

Grounding/Anchoring Yourself and Golden Bubble of Protection

Sense golden roots coming out of your feet and grounding you on the most beautiful earth. Feel it. Sense a golden bubble all around your aura; it is like extra skin—a layer of protection. It is strong and pliable but impenetrable. Feel it. This golden bubble will be activated indefinitely to protect your energy from negative people or anything environmental. Smile. Take a moment just to say thank you to your body. Your heart, your mind, your soul. Finally, open your eyes whenever you feel ready.

Review

Feel renewed; feel at peace, present and joyful. Take notes in your diary— you can read back and reflect on it all when you need to. If you are meditating in a group then allow each person the opportunity to share what magic they have experienced, remembering all the good moments. What did you feel, see, sense, or just know? What lessons can you take away from this that will help you in any way with your beautiful life journey?

Chapter Ten
Inner Child

"Unleash your inner, ageless, wonder-filled child and set her/him free, to help you reclaim boundless energy"
                                        – Carol Watson

Meet the Angel of Youth, Afriel, as you journey within to reconnect with the inner child that is you. You will discover if your inner child-self has been left, or perhaps neglected along your life's journey. Has she/he been stumped in any way and would maybe appreciate some attention; or is your inner child living deep within you in a beautiful, balanced way? Are you ready to go within?

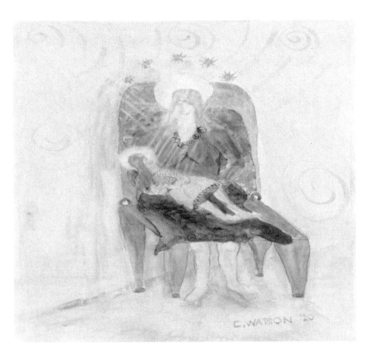

[Begin with the routine from Chapter Two first Light Body.]

At this moment, envision the beautiful Angel of Youth in her green rays and wings that represent the new leaves in spring, and are the colour of new sprouts, representing new ideas and thinking. Invite her to step forward and meet you and wrap her wings around you in a nurturing blanket. Feel her loving embrace as you stop and just feel her presence. Feel her love and gentle warmth.

Wrapped up in Afriel's wings, take a moment now to recall and visualise an old faithful friend that you had as a child. It could be a teddy bear, a doll, an action man; or a small, soft blanket. Think back now to this comforting, loving ally you had or still may even have. See it larger than life—vibrant, colourful and radiant. Does it have a name, or do you sense a feeling or colour when you think about it?

Now imagine travelling down the timeline of your life to some poignant memories you have had with this gorgeous toy or blanket in your past. How did it make you feel, what emotions did it bring you? Think about how you could harness that energy, and bring it back into your life again, even if you don't have that little ally? Contemplate what sounds were around you that you remember from that time, and how warm and comforted you felt. Allow this feeling to become a huge all singing all dancing vision that can be called upon and reanimated as your comforter whenever you are in need of it.

Ask Afriel to bring her wisdom forward now to you, as you take a moment to listen to her or perhaps even watch her show you a symbolic vision. This experience will make you understand more about how you can absorb these beautiful visions and feelings back into your life and feel that old comfort return. How good was that? Give your thanks to Afriel now.

Know that this is a safe space and no harm can come to you, and you will come back at the end feeling so much clearer and even with perhaps an epiphany about your past and how you can reclaim that nurturing time.

Now, please bring forward a memory of when you were a child that is safe for you to recall. Try and choose a memory that you are ready to face from your past, one that you might have had difficulty in resolving. Only bring what you are comfortable with, as you sit or lie down in your personal space today. Only work through remembering and bringing forward to your mind that you can handle and manage on your own.

NB. If you are processing deeper issues through a Qualified Counsellor or Coach, then do not bring any of that deeper more difficult stuff up to work through today.

The memory could be an accident or a form of loss and grief; a fall-out or telling off from a parent or guardian. Remember back to it, it is safe to do so—go back into the situation as if it was a movie screen playing in front of you now, or a radio programme playing it back as you listen to the sounds of the memory unfold. You could be more aware of how you feel and sense around you. What age were you? Know you are a witness and this is the past and cannot hurt you now in the present.

Look at how you were. You were a little vulnerable right? I want you to now picture this vision and memory that got stuck inside you going off into the distance. I want you to see it turn black and white as it shrinks smaller and smaller into insignificance. Let's work with Afriel now to open your heart and send love to this situation, the feeling or fears it had over you.

Send your younger self-love straight from your heart now and watch as Afriel surrounds this little inner child with her wings of green healing light. Watch what happens to the inner child you were. How incredible that we can go back in time and recall and even heal past memories that got stuck in us, right?

See this horrible scenario or scene distance even further from you and become almost a pinhead on the horizon. Watch it become small, lifeless, black and white; unimportant. Now work through another old situation from the past and do the same. Now one final one. How good does it feel to free yourself from these memories and sense the confidence and strength within us grow?

Think about what you learnt from those situations to turn them into a more positive experience of growth. We are all here to grow and evolve and we all understand that often the times that are the most challenging are where we learn the most once we overcome these life tests. We can often resonate with those that have gone through similar situations and so we then can bring our wisdom and support to lift that person up again. We become comforters.

Let's ask that your inner child now reveals themselves to you at the stage in life that they stopped growing *(if they did)*. Did you stop growing because of a sad death or being seriously scolded by your teacher? Call your inner child now and observe what age she or he is. Has she been stunted; is she well-groomed or dishevelled? Has she aged well? Is she quiet and withdrawn or very animated and confident with lots of energy? Open your arms to your inner child, which is you. Go to her or him and give her a huge hug.

Thank her with feeling in your heart, thank her for showing up and speaking to you now. Watch what she does, shows you or says, telepathically. Allow all of your senses to sharpen now as she becomes larger in vision, colourful, animated, bright, alive. Feel her.

Ask now what she needs to make her inner life experience with you more pleasant, rewarding and happy? Watch carefully. This is a very important moment to take notice of. Give her your thanks again and express your gratitude at her stepping forward to communicate with you. Know she will always be around if you want to take time to nurture your inner self and learn from her.

She may want more play and less seriousness, more wilderness adventures in nature with you. Be aware of the future of this beautiful soul that is you, who loves you. Offer her a gift, a love heart crystal pendant on a chain. Perhaps she needs new clothing, a grooming set, a book, a music CD, a diary, a sketch pad and coloured felt pens. Spoil her.

Ask her if there is anything she needs and if there are any words of advice she can give you to improve your life? Say thank you and goodbye for now, as she starts to fade a little. How good was this encounter? What a true blessing. You can revisit her any day or time you want and do more personal work with her if needed.

Give thanks to Afriel as her angel wings and presence also fades.

Bringing Yourself Back into Your Physical Body

It's time to return. See the physical you, standing there, arms wide open welcoming you back with a big smile. Walk towards your physical self and go around the back of you. Step into your physical body one leg at a time, like a hand slipping back into a glove. One arm, then your other arm. Bring your torso back into the body and head.

Instantly you are transported back into your room and chair. Feel the weight on your shoulders and your feet grounding you. Sense your spirit fully back and present in your body. Take some really deep breaths again; in through your mouth and out through your mouth into the lower abdomen. Now take two or three in through your nose and out through your mouth. Feel yourself in your chair now.

Grounding/Anchoring Yourself and Golden Bubble of Protection

Sense golden roots coming out of your feet and grounding you on the most beautiful earth. Feel it. Sense a golden bubble all around your aura; it is like extra skin—a layer of protection. It is strong and pliable but impenetrable. Feel it. This golden bubble will be activated indefinitely to protect your energy from negative people or anything environmental. Smile. Take a moment just to say thank you to your body. Your heart, your mind, your soul. Finally, open your eyes whenever you feel ready.

Review

Feel renewed; feel at peace, present and joyful. Take notes in your diary— you can read back and reflect on it all when you need to. If you are meditating in a group then allow each person the opportunity to share what magic they have experienced, remembering all the good moments. What did you feel, see, sense, or just know? What lessons can you take away from this that will help you in any way with your beautiful life journey? Feel touched and blessed. Smile.

Chapter Eleven
Yin and Yang

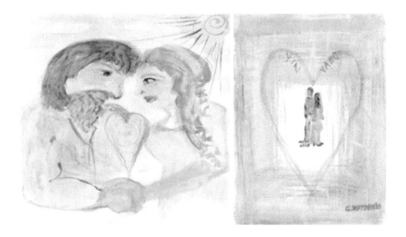

This meditation is all about observing and understanding how you care and love your inner self. It can be quite a revelatory experience and I ask you to be open-minded and open-hearted with what you observe.

[Begin by referring to your routine first in Chapter Two.]

Step out of your physical body into the light-body and onto a very white and misty long corridor with streams of potent up-light, which seems to soak into you as you walk onwards. Feel it, smell it, touch it, taste it. Through the mist ahead, you see a viewing Temple. There are steps that rise up to a platform, with a soft purple velvet large armchair. You also see a boxed and closed wicker basket to either side of the armchair. In them, you will find items you can offer your inner male and inner female as gifts when you meet them individually.

On you go, feel the buoyancy in your step and feel the lightness and wonder in your heart. As you step up and sit on your chair, take a moment to look into each basket. Both have diaries with pen and sketching pad with felt pens. You will also find a love heart necklace.

You can manifest whatever else you wish to offer the inner aspects of your own self. Perhaps a grooming kit and mirror for your inner male and a make-up bag for your inner female self. An item of clothing even. What do you want to place here? Do it with your thoughts and feelings now.

Sit and shut your eyes; reach out to your Inner Male with your whole self—your emotional heart and soul, your mind and body. Send a puff of love from your heart to him, then ask him to please reveal himself to you. He will step forward towards you out of the white mist. You may feel, sense and see him as his energy develops and grows. Your experience of him becomes stronger as he walks towards you now.

What does he look like? Is he in colour or black and white? Is he a big personality or mousy? What age is he? Has he been left behind at some time in your life and perhaps under-developed, or has he been carrying you with him aged in wisdom? Is he a spiritual man or a shallow wild man? There is no judgement here, just observation. Is he modern or old fashioned? Is he groomed and clean and well-kept or has he been a wee bit neglected? This is part of who you are as a whole so try to fully understand what you are seeing, feeling, sensing and knowing about him.

Smile and bow, feel the love, as he approaches you. Invite him to work more with you, so you can integrate him more fully into your life. You understand that with him healthy and evolved, then it will impact you and your life too. He is you. Can you tell if he is over-dominant in nature and an alpha male or under-developed in his own masculinity? Is he introverted or extroverted, has he been nurtured and cared for by you, or somehow neglected on the journey at all?

Thank him sincerely for showing himself to you, feel it in your heart. Ask him to come and take a look in one of the baskets. Let him know that you would love to give him some gifts of friendship if he is open to receiving them. He comes forward and bends down and opens the wicker basket. What is he happy to accept; what does he take and leave?

Ask him now for advice as he sits on the step at your side. Ask him how can you be more balanced on your male side? What are the over-dominant male features you have? Thank him now as he smiles back and rises and leaves. Know he is within you always, but for now, he has moved into the mist.

Invite, with a puff of love from your heart, your Inner Female self to come forward to you now. Feel it. Sense her entry as her presence becomes clearer, larger. Notice her attire, how she looks, her age, her whole energy. Is she an alpha female? Is she timid? Have you left her behind at a certain traumatic time in your life, or has she journeyed with you to the present, looking the same age as you; or is she the wise elder for you? Can you gather by her appearance whether she is spiritual or not? Feel the wonder at meeting her, if this is your first time. What a life gift. Feel it. Smile and ask her to join you. Do exactly the same as you did with your Inner Male, and show her the gifts you chose. Take as long as you need. Enjoy this incredibly special moment with her. Know this is a true blessing.

What gifts did she like and what advice did she have for you?

Your Inner Male now steps forward to take the hand of your Inner Female and takes her gently down to the water's edge just in front of you. Together they board a golden rowing boat and take off for a small Island just off in the distance. Can you see them and feel them together? They moor on the sandy bay and step off the boat by two palm trees. Your inner female lights a fire and they sit together.

Observe how they act and are comfortable in their being together? Are they a united loving couple or distant? It's time for them to return now on the wee boat. When they reach the shore they each step onto a human-sized set of golden scales into a large cup each. One at a time. When the scales are set you see if one of them is weighing heavier than the other or if they are in perfect balance.

If one is out of sync, ask how you may help them become more in alignment with the other. How can I re-balance you? Listen to the words as clear as a bell being spoken by him or her or feel it in your being. Is there any energy or word that is out of alignment, such as feelings of stubbornness, or exerting too much control? See the scales balance up as you register this and know you need to work on this aspect of yourself in order to really make the difference. If you spot that either your inner male or female is particularly out of balance, pour any virtue into the cup they stand in, and give thanks as you watch the scales balance.

It's time for them to step off the scales and return to you. See each of them re-enter your light body. They do it with effortless ease. Feel them inside you. Smile and say thank you.

It's time for you to return to your physical world now, on you go.

Bringing Yourself Back into Your Physical Body

It's time to return. See the physical you, standing there, arms wide open welcoming you back with a big smile. Walk towards your physical self and go around the back of you. Step into your physical body one leg at a time, like a hand slipping back into a glove. One arm, then your other arm. Bring your torso back into the body and head.

Instantly you are transported back into your room and chair. Feel the weight on your shoulders and your feet grounding you. Sense your spirit fully back and present in your body. Take some really deep breaths again; in through your mouth and out through your mouth into the lower abdomen. Now take two or three in through your nose and out through your mouth. Feel yourself in your chair now.

Grounding/Anchoring Yourself and Golden Bubble of Protection

Sense golden roots coming out of your feet and grounding you on the most beautiful earth. Feel it. Sense a golden bubble all around your aura; it is like an extra skin—a layer of protection. It is strong and pliable but impenetrable. Feel it. This golden bubble will be activated indefinitely to protect your energy from negative people or anything environmental. Smile. Take a moment just to say thank you to your body. Your heart, your mind, your soul. Finally, open your eyes whenever you feel ready.

Review

Feel renewed; feel at peace, present and joyful. Take notes in your diary—you can read back and reflect on all you observed and all you felt as you saw or sensed your inner aspects of self. How can you influence your life going forward now having had this encounter? What virtues or patterns can you enhance that are good ones you perhaps witnessed or felt?

For me, this was such a huge epiphany moment to actually see in my mind's eye the inner male and female of myself. I got a great understanding with clarity of how my handsome biker inner male interacts through me in this physical world. He is a huge part of my psyche. My inner male is the cool-headed, calm explorer.

He has a passion for freedom and adventure. He loves rock and blues music and as a Trinity, with my inner female and myself here in the physical we adore to dance and let our hair down. Nothing is the same now I know this part of me and welcome him into my world. I feel more whole with him in my consciousness.

My inner female self once was a fairy princess with long ringlets. Quite bohemian. I met her in meditation about fifteen years ago when I wrote this script. As a kind of wild forty-three-year-old woman, I couldn't quite relate to her and wanted a sexy biker chick woman that I resonated with. I cut her long locks and put rock chick clothes on her. I couldn't rest that night. I had to undo my makeover and apologies because this part of me enjoyed being a bright-eyed princess, innocent and gorgeous. I must say it gave a giggle to all my different Circles of friends when I shared this story before guiding them inwards to meet their own Inner male and female selves.

Fifteen years later, my inner princess has evolved at her own pace, may I add. Now I feel the Goddess, the expansive 'Cosmic-Mother' part of me, I AM. I resonate with Mary Magdalene as a huge part of my Soul-Force along with ISIS and many of the Divine Feminine Creative Principles I carry at the very core of my being. Those seeds are very much alive in me now as they can be in you if you choose to integrate them or/and, the Divine Father-God Principle.

If you are meditating in a group then allow each person the opportunity to share what magic they have experienced, remembering all the good moments. What did you feel, see, sense, or just know? What lessons can you take away from this extraordinary journey/vision? Welcome home these unacknowledged parts of you, for true parts-integration as a 'homecoming' along your beautiful life journey? Feel touched and blessed. It is an honour. Feel it. Smile.

Chapter Twelve
Archangel Michael and His
Legion of Foot Soldiers

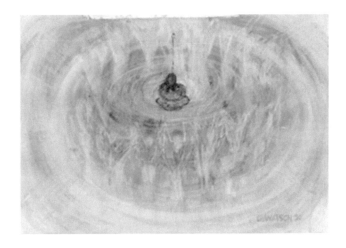

Michael is known as the most protective of all Heavenly Archangels. He protects not only humans but animals and all kingdoms. If this is the first time you meet Archangel Michael, I can assure you it will leave an indelible life-long impression on you, as he did for me the first time in around 2004 when he looked me in the eyes. It was an overwhelming, ineffable experience, stamped on my very soul. Please be ready and please enjoy. Shall we? Let's walk hand in hand together into the magnificent light of Michael.

[Begin by doing your routine from Chapter Two.]

You step out onto a sloping grassy hillside, with electric blue skies and the fluffiest white clouds overhead, and smile. Feel the earth beneath your feet, smell the aromas that you can almost taste all around you; feel the breeze in your hair and on your skin. Life is good, right?

Looking down the hill you can see an emerald green lush forest, with the most beautiful of tree species dotting along a natural earthen path into its interior, which you can just make out as a cleared area. You hear nothing but feel a tug at your tummy to go connect, go visit, meet Archangel Michael's Legion of Foot Soldiers. You sense their masculine but heavenly energy; it's animated and buoyant, happy and full of light. Head down and into your special forest. You sense the change in temperature and the musky, different smells. Be guided by the natural pathway leading you in. Enjoy.

You hear glimmers of sounds, laughter and sense animation. Send a puff of love out to these heavenly men and ask if you can step into the circle and meet Archangel Michael. You may have a vision or hear telepathic words come back to you. Feel in your gut for what they are relaying back to you. Feel it.

You must now mentally, emotionally and spiritually prepare for this magical encounter. Remember to be in awe at this phenomenal opportunity that you are being granted right here and right now. Allow your inner male and female to rise in you, and your inner child to rise and join you in this experience. Are you ready? Feel butterflies in your stomach and a swelling in your heart and an expansive opening up of your soul-self.

On you go, you have been given permission to join them. You follow the smoke rings to their small encampment. You hear the building of the noise from them and see an opening in the thick bush, allowing a glimpse of these heavenly soldiers. They are wearing silver and pale blue tunics and silver helmets. Very much like Roman soldiers but of a much higher octave of light. You can feel their vibrations.

You are close now and see the opening. You see the soldiers standing in a large circle and one catches sight of you, smiling broadly he ushers you in to join them. They have been expecting you and all the angelic men smile and welcome you. Go join them. Step into the centre of the circle as they open it up to you and bow. Feel the love and humility they have towards you. Feel your heart open so wide to them.

Bow in acknowledgement as you look eye to eye around the circle from the centre of it. Feel their enormous individual and collective beautiful and powerful presence. Smile and feel the blessing at this moment.

You sense in front of you descending light. You see it build and take shape and form—gleaming silver and sky turquoise blue, forming the silhouette of a soldiers uniform and the largest white wings. It is Archangel Michael and he is coming to meet you face to face. Feel the awe at this incredible encounter. Michael is a tall and broad warrior.

His feet touch down on the ground, a few metres from you. Far enough away for you to see all of him head to toe and look up into his sky-blue eyes; all-knowing, beautiful, protective strong eyes. Heavenly eyes. See him and bow. Feel the light from Michael pouring towards you and saturating all around the circle and out, encompassing all of the foot soldiers. Feel it. He has a Romanesque look about him and has the largest blue sword in one hand. He wears a blue cloak but also has one draped over his other arm—this is a gift for you.

Go towards Michael, you will feel as if only the two of you matter, nothing is important. Smile and bow again. You may speak to him about safety issues or about protecting your energy and aura, your home and workplace. He will listen and take time out with you. Take some minutes to really connect and communicate from the heart. He will give you some advice but also a protective gift. Give him your holy water and a crystal gift as a thank you. You know that this is the Cosmic law, we always give thanks and show our deep gratitude with the giving of gifts.

How was that? The foot soldiers now come in and close up the circle. They show you their silver shields and you feel them like a wall of protection all around you. They are there for you, as will Archangel Michael anytime you need them all. You just have to ask.

The circle opens up into a walkway now for you to exit and head back through the forest for home. Michael smiles and waves you off and the soldiers all bow and smile at you on your departure, waving as you go. It's time. You now skip through the forest, through the trees and feel the uplifting of your spirits. Your physical self is at the end of the track, looking out for you. Can you see yourself now?

Bringing Yourself Back into Your Physical Body

It's time to return. See the physical you, standing there, arms wide open welcoming you back with a big smile. Walk towards your physical self and go around the back of you. Step into your physical body one leg at a time, like a hand slipping back into a glove. One arm, then your other arm. Bring your torso back into the body and head.

Instantly you are transported back into your room and chair. Feel the weight on your shoulders and your feet grounding you. Sense your spirit fully back and present in your body. Take some really deep breaths again; in through your mouth and out through your mouth into the lower abdomen. Now take two or three in through your nose and out through your mouth. Feel yourself in your chair now.

Grounding/Anchoring Yourself and Golden Bubble of Protection

Sense golden roots coming out of your feet and grounding you on the most beautiful earth. Feel it. Sense a golden bubble all around your aura; it is like extra skin—a layer of protection. It is strong and pliable but impenetrable. Feel it. This golden bubble will be activated indefinitely to protect your energy from negative people or anything environmental. Smile. Take a moment just to say thank you to your body. Your heart, your mind, your soul. Finally, open your eyes whenever you feel ready.

Review

Many years ago, whilst living in Adelaide, Australia as a Dual Citizen (of Scotland and Australia), I came to know Archangel Michael and His Legion of Foot Soldiers. It was through guided meditation. The circle I attended for a year gave me so much creative joy and a sense of security and 'BELONGING'. I felt at home with my Meditation Teacher and the gorgeous friends of the Circle.

Meeting Michael was extraordinary for me and I hope it was for you. If not then in divine time you will experience his Presence more fully. I only ever saw Michael clearly once. It was the most personal experience. His blue, sparkling 'All-Knowing' eyes, gazed into my soul and I was mesmerised. I saw and felt His large Presence and His balanced, Heavenly, masculinity. It poured from Him and I was held in that Power. His Light is Great. You only need to call Michael once and he will be there in an instance.

I hope you have this encounter yourself. You will never forget it. I have worked daily with Archangel Michael and His Legion of Foot Soldiers to protect my aura, my home and my working Temple space where I do healing work. I feel safe and protected and I hope you did and will if you too work regularly with him.

This is a profoundly helpful meditation because as you grow in psychological maturity and develop spiritually all your senses and virtues—BECOMING more......then your light brightens. This is what it is all about. Illuminating self and ascending in consciousness so you expand and grow exponentially. However, those that are negative and feel they are lacking in themselves see your light and can want a wee bit of it to make them feel better. Therefore, protection work is absolutely vital for any growing Soul, so your auric field is protected and you feel guarded in a strong force field, a safe space.

Feel renewed; feel at peace, present and joyful. Take notes in your diary—you can read back and reflect on it all when you need to. If you are meditating in a group then allow each person the opportunity to share what magic they have experienced, remembering all the good moments. What did you feel, see, sense, or just know? What lessons can you take away from this that will help you in any way with your beautiful life journey? Feel touched and blessed. Smile.

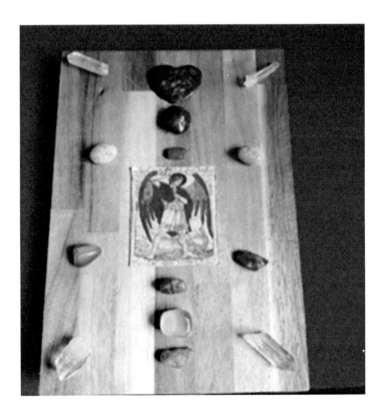

Archangel Michael depiction with crystal grid by Bridget Docherty

Chapter Thirteen
Picturing Your Future the Journey

Beautiful, spiritual friend of my heart—have you thought about what things, memories, energies or baggage you want to take with you, and who you want to take along on the journey of your life into your future? This meditation will help you focus, reflect and contemplate very deeply on what burdens or holds you down and who and allows you the space to lighten your load, giving you a joyful spring in your step. Shall we? Are you ready for some fun exploration time?

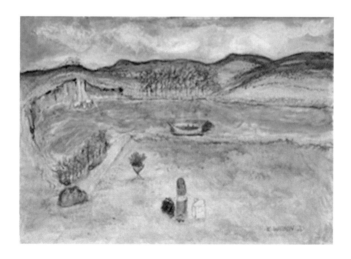

[Begin with routine from Chapter Two.]

Step out onto a grassy bank that leads down to a gentle meandering sparkling and clear river. This is your river of life. Can you see it? See the boat that is down that wee slope on the bank. It's moored up and ready for you. It has a motorised engine, so you have no work to do whatsoever apart from stepping aboard and settling in.

However, firstly, you have some work to do. Look down now to the left side of you and see a black suitcase, packed to the brim, mishappen and heavy. It's a huge suitcase. On the right side of you is a white suitcase; it looks light, with not that much in it. You can just tell without opening it up that it looks ten times lighter than the black one.

You have some work to do before getting on the boat and pushing off into your future. Next, you see a wire basket with wood sticks burning in it. This will be used to burn up things that no longer serve you. Things that tie you down to the past and burden you physically and spiritually.

Please kneel down my friend and open the big black heavy case. In this case, are pieces of clothing that reflect memories and hard challenges from the early days of your life. The thicker the texture and blacker the colour of these clothes, the older and more negative the imprint that remains embedded in you from the past. It may be a thick jumper that links you to being harshly scolded or hit by your parents, or that reflect a break-up, or a withdrawn time in your life.

Maybe even a time when you withered in yourself somehow and became quite reclusive or even angry and rebellious. Each item you lift and ponder on means something specific to you on an emotional, mental level, physical or spiritual.

There may be items from your childhood; a ruler that means harsh punishment to you, a photograph that really still grips at your heart, perhaps a school photo if you were bullied or ridiculed in any way, or a photo of a past love.

This is the time to clean up and sweep away those ugly, old, outdated, out-worn memories from your being. It's the chance to lighten and lift the load you have been carrying during your life, once and for all now. You will feel a million dollars after this meditation, I promise.

As you remove items from the suitcase and before throwing them on the fire, please do thank each one for the positive lessons it taught you about yourself. It may be how resilient you were, self-preserving, tolerant, forgiving, self-loving or accepting. Make it count. On you go.

How good did that feel to review and remove all those heavy things that no longer serve a positive purpose in your life—pretty good right? Ok, now it's time to leave that case. It is so much lighter; you have things from it you still wish to take with you right?

Now open the white case and see all the amazing items that reflect your happy moments; hugs, kindnesses, warmth and care that you have had in your life. There may be ornaments, a diary, a photo album, a treasured teddy or toy or sooky blanket in there (that is definitely coming right?) There may be gorgeous multi-coloured sparkling items or even clothes that uplift you, still, to this day, in this lovely, happy case. Are there items from school, awards, or from Guides or Scouts, or any other groups you were part of? Is there school, college or university certificates or other fabulous accolades and memories in there? Remove anything that really is no longer needed, to enable you to consolidate your cases into just the one white one.

Pat things down, roll them up to make more space and take from the black case those items that are coming into your future. There are also some new items added; one is an affirmation book full of positive statements for each day, this mediation book so you can meditate when you need help and a golden compass. This represents your spiritual life path, your reconnection to the Source, and how you will always tune in to it if you go off track.

Hidden in one of the recess pockets you'll find a selenite white shiny love heart crystal; this is your new gratitude rock. Whenever you experience something really great happen in your life, you hold your beautiful crystal and say thank you. It is a great practice to do. Now place whatever you are bringing from the black case into your lighter brighter white case. Close it and head to the golden boat.

Stepping onboard, you are prompted to think of people you are definitely bringing with you on your life journey. Call them in and let them get settled in for the ride. The boat fires up and gently takes off along the riverbanks. It speeds up and you get splashed, and everyone is laughing and happy. The boat is full of joy and energy.

Enjoy the twists and bends of the river as the boat slows and speeds up. Notice every detail and how alive you feel, how energised and light. This is a great day, right? What a blessing. You see at the left hand bend a beautiful high waterfall. It is full of sparkle and light. The boat heads for it and you are all about to float under it. It is just light—no liquid. It is a bath of white light that you can be refreshed in. It seems to flow over you and in and through your head. It's a deeply immersive light, penetrating right the way through you and your suitcase. How good does that feel?

The boat pulls out from the waterfall, fires up its engines again and zooms upriver and around the next bend; it is heading back for shore. You see yourself on the banks waving and smiling, it's time to return a whole new you. Feel it. It is time to get off the boat as it moors at the riverbank and all your loved ones fade into the mist. It's time to return to your physical self.

Bringing Yourself Back into Your Physical Body

It's time to return. See the physical you, standing there, arms wide open welcoming you back with a big smile. Walk towards your physical self and go around the back of you. Step into your physical body one leg at a time, like a hand slipping back into a glove. One arm, then your other arm. Bring your torso back into the body and head.

Instantly you are transported back into your room and chair. Feel the weight on your shoulders and your feet grounding you. Sense your spirit fully back and present in your body. Take some really deep breaths again; in through your mouth and out through your mouth into the lower abdomen. Now take two or three in through your nose and out through your mouth. Feel yourself in your chair now.

Grounding/Anchoring Yourself and Golden Bubble of Protection

Sense golden roots coming out of your feet and grounding you on the most beautiful earth. Feel it. Sense a golden bubble all around your aura; it is like extra skin—a layer of protection. It is strong and pliable but impenetrable. Feel it. This golden bubble will be activated indefinitely to protect your energy from negative people or anything environmental. Smile. Take a moment just to say thank you to your body. Your heart, your mind, your soul. Finally, open your eyes whenever you feel ready.

Review

How good and useful was that for you my beautiful friend? Feel the difference between off-loading that heavy and dark baggage. It is remarkable, isn't it? Fee the sense of actual 'space' inside your body and mind. It's almost tangible, right? How good is it to have more room inside the apartment of

'YOU' now, more room to decorate and add new fresh, uplifting additions to your future you?

Feel renewed, feel at peace, present and joyful. Take notes in your diary—you can read back and reflect on it all when you need to. If you are meditating in a group then allow each person the opportunity to share what magic they have experienced, remembering all the good moments. What did you feel, see, sense, or just know? What lessons can you take away from this that will help you in any way with your beautiful life journey? Feel touched and blessed. Smile.

Chapter Fourteen
Manifesting Abundance

[Begin with routine from Chapter Two first.]

As you step out of yourself you see a luminous white temple. It has pearlescent white steps leading up to large pearly doors, which are open. There are two spiral pillars on each side of the steps. On you go, head up them. Feel the serenity and majesty of this awesome structure. How do you feel here? There is golden misty energy emitting from the open doors, feel it drawing you towards it, and the open doors.

This temple is a chamber, a manifestation chamber for you. It is a dream chamber—head in. You will connect with the Universal energy of creation. This temple contains the energy of blessings and abundance; you will absorb and immerse yourself fully in this energy when the doors close—take a seat and get comfortable. The chamber is full of golden misty light and energy. Feel it.

The sanctuary lights switch off and the room becomes very dark; this is becoming your private viewing room. You will see a screen come up on the wall in front of you in this darkness. You will see things you are hoping to bring into your reality. Sit in quietness and stillness for now and bring to mind what you want to see and bring alive in your life. Think about your health and comfort, think about loving relationships, think about what your life's work is? What do you want to see happen for you in two to five years' time? Where are you living, how creative is your life? Know what will make your life ahead of you satisfied and fulfilled.

This is your time to manifest all your dreams, goals, and desires. When you call the first vision up on the screen in front of you, make sure you go into feeling it. Really feel you are part of this manifestation and think about how good it makes you feel. The screen will fuzz, and then change to the next picture of your dreams and desires and so on.

Take the time to really make this an incredible opportunity to manifest a phenomenal present and future for yourself. Remember to see your heart's desires also; who is in your heart, who do you want in your heart? See yourself with these loved ones and how happy and blissful you feel. Really feel it.

The room lights will slowly come back up and the golden rays swoosh around the room again. Feel it. It is time to get up and leave this chamber. Know you can revisit any time you wish to, and know that it is vital to work on manifesting all your goals regularly, so you retrain your brain with the repetition.

When your mind believes it is real, your heart does also and visualising who you have in your life and what you want in it creates your new reality. You can step out of the temple now, and walk down the steps to your physical self, who is delighted to have you back.

Bringing Yourself Back into Your Physical Body

It's time to return. See the physical you, standing there, arms wide open welcoming you back with a big smile. Walk towards your physical self and go around the back of you. Step into your physical body one leg at a time, like a hand slipping back into a glove. One arm, then your other arm. Bring your torso back into the body and head.

Instantly you are transported back into your room and chair. Feel the weight on your shoulders and your feet grounding you. Sense your spirit fully back and present in your body. Take some really deep breaths again; in through your mouth and out through your mouth into the lower abdomen. Now take two or three in through your nose and out through your mouth. Feel yourself in your chair now.

Grounding/Anchoring Yourself and Golden Bubble of Protection

Sense golden roots coming out of your feet and grounding you on the most beautiful earth. Feel it. Sense a golden bubble all around your aura; it is like extra skin—a layer of protection. It is strong and pliable but impenetrable. Feel it. This golden bubble will be activated indefinitely to protect your energy from negative people or anything environmental. Smile. Take a moment just to say

thank you to your body. Your heart, your mind, your soul. Finally, open your eyes whenever you feel ready.

Review

Is it not hugely useful to project what you want instead of constant catching up or chasing your tail. Never quite meeting those desires, or they seem to come randomly out of sync or out of time. Here you have had the opportunity to really work on what you want consciously. Focused intention and feeling into that desire is how you are going to manifest so many great things to you.

OK, you can manifest those shallow luxuries, yes new outfit, laptop, furnishings, etc but how about the creative things. The vocational new career you desperately want, the workshops to enhance your creativity, travel etc. Go deeper and really work on the new you. How you want to be received. Are you ready for the new relationship with yourself first? Perhaps you are single and always hoping for a new man, a new woman, a better relationship etc.

Remember words like 'I need, I want, can I, could I' do not manifest anything, they leave you needing and wanting. Words are powerful my friend, use them wisely. Consciously say your affirmations with clear intent as if you already HAVE received what you ask for. Thank you's are part of it.

Smile.

Chapter Fifteen
Snowball Effect

We have all heard of this expression, right? We all know how it can cause issues in our lives when sometimes we don't even know we are doing something repetitively in a negative way. So the snowball effect really is an accumulation of events that get out of hand and impact our life some meaningful, and some negative or even harmful. This is a very useful and healing meditation to recognise life patterns and how you have given things wings in a positive way but also in a negative way during our lifetime. We all can harness the positive patterns, through recognition and influencing them along with the more stubborn or challenging ones.

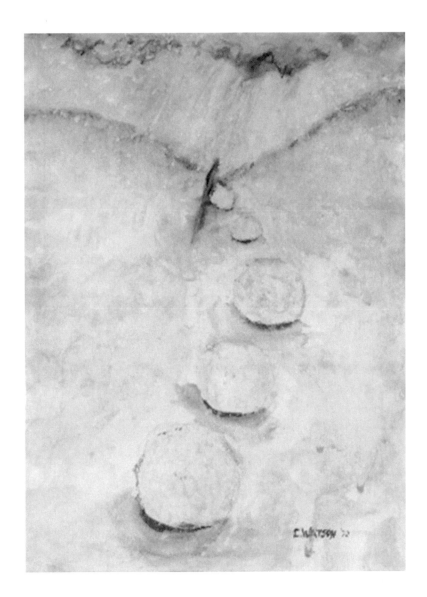

Imagine lying in a very comfortable bed as you begin slipping down the timeline of your life, back down the years, one year at a time, until you reach certain pivotal landmarks.

Remember as a little one, a baby, or a wee child, when something scary happened to you. Perhaps it was when you were in the paddling pool or bathtub and you slipped under the water when your parent or guardian wasn't looking and the panic you felt was horrendous. You believed at that moment your life was over. Did this happen to you? It is essential to not let memories like this snowball.

It could have been a time when a dog chased you, barking like a rabid beast, terrifying you. It could be a large spider that dropped on your arm or head and was so scary you have been terrified of them ever since.

Perhaps you lost someone close, who was so young and left well before their time, and you put thought into your mind that you would not live past that age yourself as I once did with my Father as he died prematurely at the age of only forty-five. I embedded an imprint with my consciousness and by working on myself, reviewing negative patterns I was able to address this imprint.

We all put imprints into our consciousness and now it's a chance to clear the negative ones or at least to begin this process. Visit the scenario, but remember you are only an observer. You are looking at this from a distant viewpoint. It is a place of higher perspective, with no emotion attached to it. This perspective allows you to witness the memory without the attachment to it, without the fear and without the feeling it always caused you in the past.

Watch how real it was and acknowledge it, send a loving comforting blanket and embrace yourself. Soothe yourself. Explain that you have nothing to fear now and then release this memory. Observe how you gave it wings and if it was a fear of drowning how it grew into a fear of being submerged and water in general and how it really impacted your life.

Or if it is a fear of spiders notice how this sadly snowballed into a real fear of dogs and then horses and then other animals. Visit and work through one— two of your phobias or fears and see in the timeline how you gave it wings and it grew. All along comfort your inner self. The frightened self.

How empowering was that? Great right? Now let's go and see down the timeline an amazing snowball scenario from how it happened to how it has influenced and helped your life expand and stretch beyond all imagining. This could be fear of leaving your home and comfort of your immediate area you lived in as a youth, then district and town, and how through facing your insecurities about it you adventured further afield bit by bit, then into the wider country and then into other countries.

Think about how amazing it felt when you moved to another location or even country. How it astonished you to return to your family home and meet old neighbourhood friends who never ever ventured anywhere and who still talked about childhood as if these are their only memories. You then see how huge your life is; expansive, bigger, happier even maybe more whole and fulfilling. It could be about the study and going into an occupation you never in a million years felt you could do and how through focus, study and determination your true grit is or has paid off.

See the snowball effect it has caused, you could be doing an advanced study to get more recognition or could be sharing what you know, look at one or two positive things that snowballed for you from your efforts.

[Begin with your routine from Chapter Two first.]

I want you to step out of your warm bed or chair, into the outdoor wilderness. A snow-capped mountain is opposite you and a thick foot of snow covers a sloping meadow right in front of you. Time to bring your inner child out to play. Feel the icy cold as the sun beats down on you. You are wrapped up and you have thick warm thermal gloves on. Go create some magic. Find a pile of snow and build a snowball. You will run with it down the hill as it grows bigger and bigger. Enjoy.

Bringing Yourself Back into Your Physical Body

It's time to return. See the physical you, standing there, arms wide open welcoming you back with a big smile. Walk towards your physical self and go around the back of you. Step into your physical body one leg at a time, like a hand slipping back into a glove. One arm, then your other arm. Bring your torso back into the body and head.

Instantly you are transported back into your room and chair. Feel the weight on your shoulders and your feet grounding you. Sense your spirit fully back and present in your body. Take some really deep breaths again; in through your mouth and out through your mouth into the lower abdomen. Now take two or three in through your nose and out through your mouth. Feel yourself in your chair now.

Grounding/Anchoring Yourself and Golden Bubble of Protection

Sense golden roots coming out of your feet and grounding you on the most beautiful earth. Feel it. Sense a golden bubble all around your aura; it is like extra skin—a layer of protection. It is strong and pliable but impenetrable. Feel it. This golden bubble will be activated indefinitely to protect your energy from negative people or anything environmental. Smile. Take a moment just to say

thank you to your body. Your heart, your mind, your soul. Finally, open your eyes whenever you feel ready.

Review

I had implanted a thought that grew wings and then became a snowball I rolled down my imaginary downward hill every day I woke up for almost ten years. My implanted negative thought was about my Dad who died at the age of forty-five. Young right! Yes, he was ill and we knew he was suffering. However, it came as such as shock to lose him so suddenly.

From the following day upon awakening, I had implanted a negative thought about life not being worth living without him. Every morning I woke to these thoughts and so they became embedded and like a snowball got bigger and more scary each day. It took me ten years and therapy to realise I could change it and I did.

I have never had that recurring awful thought again since doing focused work on it. Just as you can with your repeated negative pattern. It could be a phobia about a mouse, a spider, your weight, anything. Change the script you tell yourself and change for the better.

Feel renewed; feel at peace, present and joyful. Take notes in your diary—you can read back and reflect on it all when you need to. If you are meditating in a group then allow each person the opportunity to share what magic they have experienced, remembering all the good moments. What did you feel, see, sense, or just know? What lessons can you take away from this that will help you in any way with your beautiful life journey? Feel touched and blessed, smile.

Chapter Sixteen
The Healing Cabin

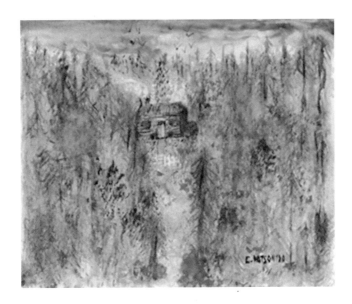

[Begin with your routine from Chapter Two.]

You step out onto a high wild meadow with the sun high in the sky and a warm, gentle breeze blowing through your hair and kissing your skin. You think, *'this is a good place to be!'* You see an emerald forest at the foot of this sloping meadow and a trail that leads into the interior. You can see that there is a cabin in the centre of this dense beautiful forest as you see a ring of smoke dancing through the air from its fire. Head down to the forest and head into the interior towards that magical, secret healing cabin.

That is what it is. On you go. As you reach the entrance leading in, you can see the trail; green fairy lights are hanging off the branches on all the trees along the path. You see a darting light, a sparkle here and there; what do you see or sense? It is the fairies.

They will lead you towards your secret cabin. On you go, enjoy this experience. Let your inner child come out to play. Observe all the various colours of the trees, as autumn is in full bloom. Red, oranges, ever-greens, yellows, purples. How magnificent.

You see a hint of the cabin through the trees, way up ahead—head for it. Brushing through some bushes you catch the cabin in all its magnificence, surrounded by a multitude of coloured trees behind it. You notice a tiny, cobbled, winding path that leads to a white small picket fence and gate. Flower boxes sit near the cabin making it a strikingly beautiful setting to behold. You can smell the peat fire and see the green door of the cabin inviting you in. On you go. It's been made ready for you. Go to the door and turn the handle and step inside.

As you step inside you are surrounded by gentle spa music playing with sweet guitar tunes and warm deep mist. Feel the heat from the peat fire as you go towards it. There is a rocking chair with a white robe and towel with white slippers sitting on it. It is for you. Turn around now and you see the most exquisite small, liquid green healing pool or plunge pool at the other end of the room.

Steps lead down into the warming fizzing waters. You can smell essential oils in the air rising from it; lavender, lemon, peppermint and mandarin. A cocktail of phenomenal scents. You can feel the essence of this green water, and you know it is a deeply healing pool.

Change and place your clothes on the rocking horse and take some steps down and into the luxurious spa pool. Immerse yourself in this energy. It feels tingly on the skin and powerful in a soft and gorgeous sort of way. There is a deep tunnel in the pool that leads to the outside if you are wanting to dive down and explore. It is your time. Enjoy for as long as you like.

The door near the peat fire is opening and you are now welcome to invite a loved one from the other side. It can be anyone you have missed and wish to reconnect within this beautiful healing space and pool. It could be a sibling, child, partner, parent or grandparent. The choice is both yours and theirs.

Call their name and say these words "in accordance with your own Divine Will, would like to step through the veil and join me for a little while? If so, then please step through the dimensional door now." Smile. This is your time to really savour this magical and special moment. Who came to meet you? How do they look? Invite them to step into the pool and join you. Take as long as you like to reconnect; talk, play, share, have fun. How good does this feel? How blessed do you feel to have this moment?

It's time now for your loved one to leave the pool and enter back through the dimensional doorway. Say your goodbyes and wave them off, till the next time.

It's now time for you to exit the healing pool and dry off at the gorgeous warm fire and dress. In your pockets are the New Earth elixir, holy water and a rose quartz crystal love heart. Throw the love heart in the pool and spray it with the elixir as a little gratitude blessing. Life is good. Smile. It's time to leave the cabin and head back through the forest for home. Follow the fairy trail of green lights, swing off the ropes if you want or skip along the trail, back to the entrance of the forest.

You see a fairy at the entrance fluttering and sparkling. She has a little gift for you. On you go. What is it? Give your thanks. Bless the fairy with your elixir.

As you leave the forest you see the physical you, standing there.

Bringing Yourself Back into Your Physical Body

It's time to return. See the physical you, standing there, arms wide open welcoming you back with a big smile. Walk towards your physical self and go around the back of you. Step into your physical body one leg at a time, like a hand slipping back into a glove. One arm, then your other arm. Bring your torso back into the body and head.

Listen to 'The Healing Cabin' under my name, Carol Watson, if you wish to hear my voice. https://youtu.be/CFFanuJWxLac

Instantly you are transported back into your room and chair. Feel the weight on your shoulders and your feet grounding you. Sense your spirit fully back and present in your body. Take some really deep breaths again; in through your mouth and out through your mouth into the lower abdomen. Now take two or three in through your nose and out through your mouth. Feel yourself in your chair now.

Grounding/Anchoring Yourself and Golden Bubble of Protection

Sense golden roots coming out of your feet and grounding you on the most beautiful earth. Feel it. Sense a golden bubble all around your aura; it is like extra skin—a layer of protection. It is strong and pliable but impenetrable. Feel it. This golden bubble will be activated indefinitely to protect your energy from negative people or anything environmental. Smile. Take a moment just to say thank you to your body. Your heart, your mind, your soul. Finally, open your eyes whenever you feel ready.

Review

My friend, this is such a useful meditation to regularly undertake, if you need some healing or calm. It is, and has been, so well-loved by the Rainbow Path Tribe over the years and myself. I have found it nourishing and immersive and I have met my Dad and my Beloved Twin-Flame in the healing pool, which has been so love-enhancing for me. You may have met a gorgeous loved one yourself in the pool, a deceased family member or your partner, or a child if you have one. It is like having a sooky blanket to enfold you in love and warmth and I hope you get lots of pleasure from it each time you revisit this meditation.

Feel renewed; feel at peace, present and joyful. Take notes in your diary—you can read back and reflect on it all when you need to. If you are meditating in a group then allow each person the opportunity to share what magic they have experienced, remembering all the good moments. What did you feel, see, sense, or just know? What lessons can you take away from this that will help you in any way with your beautiful life journey? Feel touched and blessed. Smile.

Chapter Seventeen
The Gardener

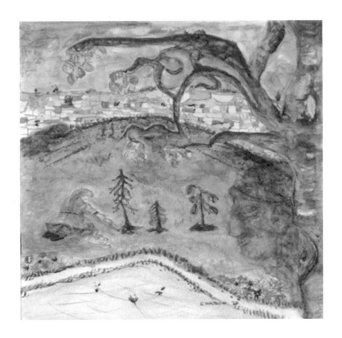

[Begin first with your routine from Chapter Two.]

As you step out of your physical body, step onto a rickety windy leafy path that is lined with trees. There are hedges and trees lining both sides of your private path. It is a mystical, secret path; your path. Enjoy the stroll downhill as you listen to birds chirping and butterflies fluttering by. See the rainbow rays of light stream through the tree canopy and onto your beautiful path. How do you feel? Isn't it a good place to be?

As you stroll on through this winding rickety path, you see at the bottom a high stone wall with ivy growing up it and large golden metal gates, which are open. Can you see it? There is a special gardener, a guide waiting on you, to welcome you into this secret, heavenly garden. On you go.

You both bow and acknowledge one another with a big lovely smile and he ushers you in with a wave of his hand. He has been expecting you. As you step into the magical garden you are hit with the aromas of the most exquisite orchids and lilies, roses and wild herbs. You feel the atmosphere, which is incredibly light and beautiful, bringing you a sense of joy. It seems to embrace you as the colour and smells seem to soak into you too. You sense a misty fountain close by and feel its cooling spray. Can you see it? It is so pretty and enchanting.

The Gardener beckons you to follow him and gives you a little trowel and small golden sack with golden seeds in it. He tells you as you walk with him towards the back wall that you will be on your knees for this job. You will be doing some weeding. Weeding of your own issues. Things that are niggling you or buried deep down.

This is a healing garden you see, and you will feel so much better after doing this wonderful, useful work. He points to the weedy patch at the back wall with a wire basket that has been lit and is now burning. You are informed that you can throw the old stuck weeds into it as you work. He tells you that you are burning the old patterns, hurts and pains away as you uproot your own weeds inside you.

Each weed you will now look at and begin removing. He asks you to get down on your hands and knees by this patch of yours and he leaves you alone. Take your hand trowel and call forward into your mind the first issue that you'd love to get rid of. Is it about work or money worries, a relationship that is disturbing you? Where you live? Take your time with grabbing hold of each weed and start to haul it up as you dig.

You will understand just how deep or shallow this particular issue is by the depth and spread of the roots and by how tough it is to uproot. Take as long as you need to do this work, one issue at a time until you feel you've exhausted all the things that have upset you of late. How does it feel? Good right? Now toss them all on the fire and see them frazzle and burn away.

Take the golden sack and spread your seeds on the ground and think now of the beautiful things you want to have in your life. Each seed will represent an area of manifestation you want to work on. Remember to make sure it is well planted and use the watering can close by to water each seed. When you are done with planting all of them, stand up and water them all.

As you do you begin to see the seeds sprout into saplings, popping through the rich soil and stretching upwards. See the tiny leaves and stems strengthen and grow bigger and taller as you watch. How does it make you feel? Now take the magical holy elixir from your pocket and spray the plants with the new earth energy.

It's time to head out of the secret garden, but firstly, you can go take a ribbon from the branch near the big oak tree and think of something you are really grateful for in your life. Tie the ribbon on the big oak tree as you give your thanks. See all the colourful ribbons blowing in the breeze of this big happy tree. Head back towards the Gardener who is waiting to say farewell to you at the gate.

Thank the Gardener for this experience and offer him a lovely crystal love heart as a way of showing your gratitude for today. Ask him if he has a personal message for you right now, one that you can take on board for your life—something wise and helpful. Listen to what he shares, or watch what he does. Say thank you once more. After your goodbyes, you leave the garden and head back up the crooked pathway.

You see your physical self, there, at the very top of the hill, smiling broadly, welcoming you back.

Bringing Yourself Back into Your Physical Body

It's time to return. See the physical you, standing there, arms wide open welcoming you back with a big smile. Walk towards your physical self and go around the back of you. Step into your physical body one leg at a time, like a hand slipping back into a glove. One arm, then your other arm. Bring your torso back into the body and head.

Instantly you are transported back into your room and chair. Feel the weight on your shoulders and your feet grounding you. Sense your spirit fully back and present in your body. Take some really deep breaths again; in through your mouth and out through your mouth into the lower abdomen. Now take two or three in through your nose and out through your mouth. Feel yourself in your chair now.

Grounding/Anchoring Yourself and Golden Bubble of Protection

Sense golden roots coming out of your feet and grounding you on the most beautiful earth. Feel it. Sense a golden bubble all around your aura; it is like extra skin—a layer of protection. It is strong and pliable but impenetrable. Feel it. This golden bubble will be activated indefinitely to protect your energy from negative people or anything environmental. Smile. Take a moment just to say thank you to your body. Your heart, your mind, your soul. Finally, open your eyes whenever you feel ready.

Review

This works as a treat for manifesting your goals and dreams. I have loved this one as have the Rainbow Path Tribe over the years, as I hope you will enjoy it too and use it alongside your affirmations and Picturing Your Future meditation. They all work as a tool kit for the Great future YOU.

Feel renewed; feel at peace, present and joyful. Take notes in your diary—you can read back and reflect on it all when you need to. If you are meditating in a group then allow each person the opportunity to share what magic they have experienced, remembering all the good moments. What did you feel, see, sense, or just know? What lessons can you take away from this that will help you in any way with your beautiful life journey? Feel touched and blessed. Smile.

Chapter Eighteen
Meeting Your Animal Guide(s)

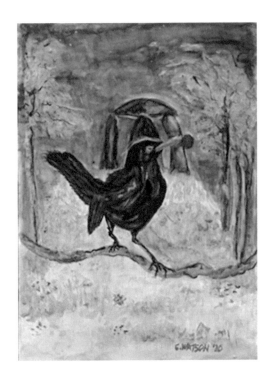

[Begin with your routine from Chapter Two.]

Step into a sunlit, evergreen magical forest track with all of your favourite species of medicinal plants and trees. Smell the fresh air, which is oxygen-filled and full of light and excitement. Head into the trail; skip, sing, bring out your inner child, have fun. Ahead of you, you see a hollowed-out massive yew tree. It is a mystical and magical tree that is a link between worlds and is often found in graveyards. This divine guardian tree invites you to step into its auric field.

Sense this energy four metres from you, go closer, two metres and you feel it intensify, immersed in its beautiful musky alive energy. Step into the hollow in the trunk and feel the cool musk of the inner sanctum of the tree. Feel the earth beneath your feet, feel part of this ancient being. You see in the dark an old wooden rail leading down into the underworld.

It is safe to go and meet your Animal Guide in this other realm. I will guide you back safely at the end. Feel the smoothness and cool of the wood, soak up the smells and energy of this living deity. Downwards in a spiral, you go. You see a glimmer of light out the other side of the tree tunnel.

You smell the cool air and sense the water droplets in the air of a small loch ahead, out the other side. Step out into this small valley with hills and trees snuggling in a small jet-black loch. See the path, you are going to walk all the way around it and back into this tree tunnel at the end. However, firstly, my friend, you are going to meet your animal guide, to guide you.

On you go—walk along that lovely golden path and tune in to your surroundings, ask that your master animal guide (or Totem, as she is known by some cultures) come to meet you. Smile and send a puff of love out to this Teacher Guide. She will be picking up your scent; as you walk, continue to call out to her or him. What animal do you sense as you walk—do you have any images of her in your mind? Look out for her, who do you see? Notice everything she does and shows you, as it is all significant and useful wisdom to you, and your current life, and will help you harness her beautiful energy to help you.

Tune in, shut your eyes when you can to really immerse yourself in this experience. Ask her to communicate through telepathy, mind-to-mind words, and to show you images. Enjoy. This is your time. Take as long as you like.

Give your thanks. Offer her a beautiful blessing of the New Earth holy elixir spray and put a gorgeous love heart pendant on her neck as a sign of your total gratitude and humility. She will walk with you around the loch, on you go. Enjoy one another's company. What can you learn from this species that you can integrate into your own life?

Is there another Animal Guide that wishes to meet and work with you? Look out for another visitor. Know that these guides will remain with you till you need a new Animal Totem/Helper. Enjoy the sights and sounds and smells of this mystical land of Scotland. Feel it.

It is four billion years old; the oldest rock strata on the planet. Feel the energy of the land as you walk around the other side and back for the tree tunnel. Has any other animal come forward with a message? Give thanks if it has. Bless it also and give it a gift of thanks. It is vitally important to give thanks for everything we receive.

You now reach the tree roots and the tunnel that will return you back to your own realm. Thank your animal Guides. Give a hug and wave as you enter the dark spiral tunnel. Know you can connect with them anytime you wish. How blessed do you feel today? How amazing right?

As you head back up the dark tree tunnel, you reach the hollow floor of the Yew. Spray this inner body of the tree and the outside of it with the New Earth holy water. Go leave a love heart crystal in its centre as a show of deep love and gratitude to this wise one. Say thank you. Wave this tree off. Head back along the track.

Bringing Yourself Back into Your Physical Body

It's time to return. See the physical you, standing there, arms wide open welcoming you back with a big smile. Walk towards your physical self and go around the back of you. Step into your physical body one leg at a time, like a hand slipping back into a glove. One arm, then your other arm. Bring your torso back into the body and head.

Instantly you are transported back into your room and chair. Feel the weight on your shoulders and your feet grounding you. Sense your spirit fully back and present in your body. Take some really deep breaths again; in through your mouth and out through your mouth into the lower abdomen. Now take two or three in through your nose and out through your mouth. Feel yourself in your chair now.

Grounding/Anchoring Yourself and Golden Bubble of Protection

Sense golden roots coming out of your feet and grounding you on the most beautiful earth. Feel it. Sense a golden bubble all around your aura; it is like extra skin—a layer of protection. It is strong and pliable but impenetrable. Feel it. This golden bubble will be activated indefinitely to protect your energy from negative people or anything environmental.

Smile. Take a moment just to say thank you to your body. Your heart, your mind, your soul. Finally, open your eyes whenever you feel ready.

Review

How can you incorporate your Animal Totem into your life? What did you learn, really learn from what she or he showed you? Take notes in your diary—you can read back and reflect on it all when you need to. I have had many different two- and four-legged animals or mythical guides over the past say eighteen years. The right one comes when you meditate and ask. They will bring just the right energy, wisdom and messages to help you if you need a hand.

If you are meditating in a group then allow each person the opportunity to share what magic they have experienced, remembering all the good moments. What did you feel, see, sense, or just know? What lessons can you take away from this that will help you in any way with your beautiful life journey? Feel touched and blessed. Smile.

Chapter Nineteen
Dolphin and Whales

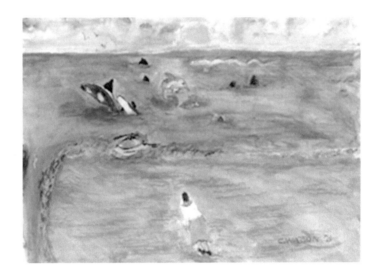

[Begin with your routine from Chapter Two.]

As you step out of your physical self, you step into the warm sand. Feel your feet and toes sinking into it as you look at this beautiful beach in front of you. Observe the flow and ebb of the turquoise sea, foamy bubbles and seaweed on the shore. You see a fabulous picnic blanket ahead on the white sand; go take a wander and take a seat on it. How good do you feel here?

You also spot a tiny golden boat with oars sitting on the shore, close to the picnic blanket. This is your boat. You will be able to head down and climb on board and be rowed out a little bit into the sea. You are going to meet either some dolphin friends or an Orca whale. Perhaps both. So when you are ready, head down to it and step onboard.

Feel the boat be gently guided out into the water as if held by the love of the ocean. It is so safe and calm and the sky is just gorgeous. How do you feel here? Smile and say thank you for your blessed life. How fortunate you are in this blissful moment. Feel it.

Smell the salt air as you spot a fin on the water, just a little way out. Can you see it? What is the creature you see pop her head up out of the deep? Send a message out to her to connect. Do this now. Can you see her? What is she doing? Watch her antics. She swims towards your boat to connect and communicate with you.

This is your time. You can even slip into the water and join her if you feel you can. It is up to you. This is your time to really enjoy this wonderful experience. The creature now throws a gift onto your boat. A precious keepsake that will remind you of this encounter. Give your thanks. You have spotted a rainbow glitter softball on the wee boat. Toss it over as a gift to your new friend and send her your love and gratitude.

It's time to return to shore. The boat manoeuvres around and is now heading for the shore, as the creature dives into the depths again. What lessons have you learned from this amazing experience? How can you integrate these lessons into your daily life?

You see the physical you on the shore now waving at you.

Bringing Yourself Back into Your Physical Body

It's time to return. See the physical you, standing there, arms wide open welcoming you back with a big smile. Walk towards your physical self and go around the back of you. Step into your physical body one leg at a time, like a hand slipping back into a glove. One arm, then your other arm. Bring your torso back into the body and head.

Instantly you are transported back into your room and chair. Feel the weight on your shoulders and your feet grounding you. Sense your spirit fully back and present in your body. Take some really deep breaths again; in through your mouth and out through your mouth into the lower abdomen. Now take two or three in through your nose and out through your mouth. Feel yourself in your chair now.

Grounding/Anchoring Yourself and Golden Bubble of Protection

Sense golden roots coming out of your feet and grounding you on the most beautiful earth. Feel it. Sense a golden bubble all around your aura; it is like extra skin—a layer of protection. It is strong and pliable but impenetrable. Feel it. This golden bubble will be activated indefinitely to protect your energy from negative people or anything environmental. Smile. Take a moment just to say thank you to your body. Your heart, your mind, your soul. Finally, open your eyes whenever you feel ready.

Review

Feel renewed; feel at peace, present and joyful. Take notes in your diary— you can read back and reflect on it all when you need to. If you are meditating in a group then allow each person the opportunity to share what magic they have experienced, remembering all the good moments. What did you feel, see, sense, or just know? What lessons can you take away from this, which will help you in any way with your beautiful life journey? Feel touched and blessed.

For me, I have a deep affinity to the Orca. I have ridden on His back and felt the world resonance of His call. Orca the whale is outstanding in my eyes. I feel so loved up with the spirit and consciousness of this alive creature. What millions of people do not understand, all creatures all animate things in nature are conscious and alive and can communicate.

They all communicate in symbolism, pictures in your mind. Angels, archangels, ascended masters all communicate this way too. It is such a life-enhancing journey to realise this and integrate all of their teachings, support and love into your life. It is a deep blessing. Smile. Practice it daily for no reason whatsoever. You will notice the difference in your life just by breathing and smiling consciously.

Chapter Twenty
Crop Circle

On 25 May 2020, at Uffington, Wiltshire, England, UK, a crop circle was formed in the cornfield, beneath the hill where the chalk-white horse is carved, in acknowledgement of the National Health Service (NHS) workers of the UK during the COVID-19 Pandemic. These are sacred geometric, circular or pictorial representations of humanity's consciousness. You may decide who they are formed by through meditation. Enjoy!

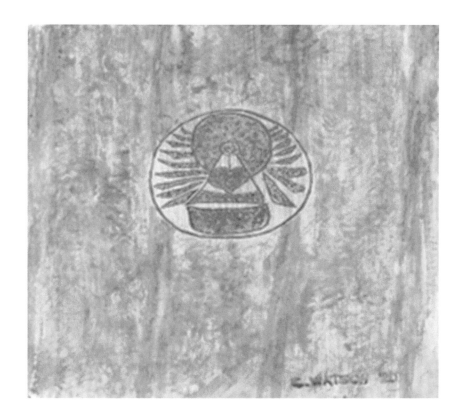

[Begin with your routine from Chapter Two.]

Imagine stepping out onto an English cornfield, below the ancient white horse chalk monument, which was chiselled in clay up on the hillside above. Take a small cushion and blanket in your rucksack on your back for later and some water. Take in the gently rolling golden cornfields, grassy landscape and sweeping soft hills of this ancient land. Sense all the sacred sites' magnetic energies, especially Stonehenge, Avebury stones, Glastonbury Tor and the Chalice Well. Feel the connection between you and these sites.

Go up the side of Uffington Hill, where the white horse image lies in the landscape so you are elevated to observe a magnificent light show. On you go. Find a comfortable spot to sit down in the grass watching the cornfield below you.

Look at the health of all the stalks and the rows that are created by the farmer's tractor. Shades of green lines and golden brown and yellow stalks stand upright in rows, with their feathery heads on display. The beginning of twilight descends over you, like a blanket of rich deep velvet warmth. The sparkling stars seem to be brought down from the heavens too as if you are surrounded by sparkle. Feel it. Watch how the moon reflects on the stalks on the cornfield below.

The cornfield is pitch black. Feel the energy building in the air. You can sense something extraordinary is about to happen. The atmosphere feels charged with electromagnetic energy. You feel the air fizz, tingle. Tune in.

You feel excitement build from your tummy upwards. You ask that your Higher Self descends to experience this with you and call upon your inner child and inner male/female self to join you more consciously for this memorable encounter.

You feel the air move and concentrate in circular formations. Three or four little tiny orbs of energy, the size of your hand, become clear as they grow in the light; building up into strong golden-white glowing globes, over the cornfield below. Can you see it? Watch carefully as they swirl like dancing ballerinas. They swirl over to the opposite patch of land that seems to be forming into a circular pattern. The energy from these beautiful orbs of consciousness becomes more concentrated and focused.

Is this the Watchers or Great Spirit at work? Is this humankind's collective consciousness mirroring what is going on with the collective of humanity, as the crop circles always seem to mirror events or affirm/confirm what we are going through or gone through with pictorial and mandala images in the crops? See how precision focused the orbs are, as the lines and circles they are forming are light white laser light in the dark night.

On 25 May 2020, during the COVID-19 world pandemic lockdown, the National Health Service in the UK (NHS) worked so hard for all those infected people. It is this crop circle you are going to see form. You see the heart in it take shape and nine lines up each side of the circular, forming the picture above. (See my depiction I painted in watercolour).

The work is finished and the orbs disappear as quickly as they came.

It is as if the curtains are being drawn back from a theatrical performance; the purple velvet sky and stars rise from the scene and dawn breaks. See the mist sitting over the land as you gather your things and head down to the crop circle. Ask The Watchers' permission to step into this landscape painting in corn. As you do, feel how charged the earth beneath your feet is and sense the energy still circulating through the mandala artwork. Look how no corn stalk is broken; only bent or twisted to shape. It is miraculous. No human hand could produce this. It is exceptional.

Go to the love heart image, representing the love we have of the health service not only in the UK but wherever you live. Not only the health service globally but to all those who have been there to help when you are unwell and then lie down as the mist rises. Feel yourself descend into that love, as depicted by the corn love heart. Go sit in it and feel the ripples of love vibrating outwards wide and far and also trip up your body and aura in pulses of rippling love vibrations. You feel like you are sinking into the earth and then rising, levitating off the ground almost.

You are surrounded by a fizz of light and love as the mist rises. Feel held in this very sacred space. Smile. Take time to enjoy and then give thanks for all the times you were tended to, loved and cared for. Say thank you! When you are ready, rise and lay a love heart crystal in this heart centre and feel it vibrate outwards and dissipate like the mist. Take the New Earth elixir, holy water from your pocket and bless the heart, feel it expand outwards in rippling cosmic waves.

The waves touch the whole of the crop circle and The Creators of this magnificent mandala to life. Now stand there and ask that the Venus energy rises from the earth below your feet, which is due to rise from the inner planes on 25 June. Feel the essence of the Divine Feminine planet, all her power, rising through the heart of this magnificent crop circle and rising upwards through you, from your feet into the sky and heavens above. Feel it. Smile and say thank you.

Ask the watchers to show you a symbol or image, or to give you words revealing what you may take from and share of this crop formation. I want you to also now see an upright and inverted pyramid, a diamond descend from above, from The Watchers and then descend through you. This symbol represents the balance of both male and female polarities within us but also the love from above and also below. Now, when you are ready, gently leave the circle.

Bringing Yourself Back into Your Physical Body

It's time to return. See the physical you, standing there, arms wide open welcoming you back with a big smile. Walk towards your physical self and go around the back of you. Step into your physical body one leg at a time, like a hand slipping back into a glove. One arm, then your other arm. Bring your torso back into the body and head.

Instantly you are transported back into your room and chair. Feel the weight on your shoulders and your feet grounding you. Sense your spirit fully back and present in your body. Take some really deep breaths again; in through your mouth and out through your mouth into the lower abdomen. Now take two or three in through your nose and out through your mouth. Feel yourself in your chair now.

Grounding/Anchoring Yourself and Golden Bubble of Protection

Sense golden roots coming out of your feet and grounding you on the most beautiful earth. Feel it. Sense a golden bubble all around your aura; it is like extra skin—a layer of protection. It is strong and pliable but impenetrable. Feel it. This golden bubble will be activated indefinitely to protect your energy from negative people or anything environmental. Smile. Take a moment just to say thank you to your body. Your heart, your mind, your soul. Finally, open your eyes whenever you feel ready.

Review

Feel renewed; feel at peace, present and joyful. Take notes in your diary—you can read back and reflect on it all when you need to. If you are meditating in a group then allow each person the opportunity to share what magic they have experienced, remembering all the good moments. What did you feel, see, sense, or just know? What lessons can you take away from this that will help you in any way with your beautiful life journey? Feel touched and blessed.

My two sisters were blessed, my friend to once witness in the South of England, near Glastonbury the formation of a Crop Circle as it happened. They saw lights and orbs zigzagging and moving in sync over the crop field and avenues, rows, circles and shapes began to form. It was a mind-blowing experience they shared with me. I did feel a little envious I must say.

I do believe there are Beings or Watchers who map out our human endeavours to show us where we are at with these crop circles. I feel it is reassuring to know that the 'Un-seen' realm interacts with us. This is only my opinion and may not be yours. I wanted to share that with you.

Smile.

Chapter Twenty-One
Heart-Hearth

"Today, see if you can stretch your heart and expand your love so that it touches not only those to whom you can give it easily but also to those who need it so much."

– Greek Philosopher, Aristotle, Born 385 BC

[Begin with your routine from Chapter Two first Light Body.]

For this experience, you will remain fully present in your body. Visualise your beautiful big puffy heart, full of life, energy and vitality. A happy heart. Smile into your beautiful Sacred, Sweet-Heart. Say I SEE YOU. Thank your heart. Tell it 'I love and I value you'. Smile. Feel the warmth of your smile and glow light up your heart chambers and make it swell with love.

Breathe with the heart's beat; connect to the rhythm that keeps you alive on this New Earth. Now take your consciousness closer towards your heart and sense yourself merging. As you become part of your heart, you see a vision of a rocking chair and a beautiful ornate heart in a cosy little den—this is your hearts-hearth. Feel the warmth and intimacy of this sacred chamber. This is your special place. Look at the crackling sticks and lumps of black coal in the fire. Meditate on the colours of the flames; reds, oranges, yellows and white flames, dancing and illuminating your wee room, your sacred sanctuary.

What would you like to frazzle up from your past in this transformative, heavenly fire? Call anything forward now and see it begin to crackle and frazzle away. Think of anything you want to add passion and fire that drives your imagination and makes you come alive. See all these inspirations light up as little dancing flames and globes of light in the fire. How good was that?

Now acknowledge the Golden, Sovereign Heart of yours, known as your Higher Heart—the Spiritual non-physical large heart that sits in the centre of your chest. Speak to it, ask for advice and information about anything you wish. Smile. Now when you are finished, give your thanks.

Imagine linking hearts with all your new companion Rainbow Path Tribe and sending a puff of love to them all and to the global community of 'Light-Workers'. Smile. Feel and know you are part of a beautiful and very special family. You are loved. Feel it. Smile and say thank you.

Bringing Yourself Back into Your Physical Body

It's time to return. See the physical you, standing there, arms wide open welcoming you back with a big smile. Walk towards your physical self and go around the back of you. Step into your physical body one leg at a time, like a hand slipping back into a glove. One arm, then your other arm. Bring your torso back into the body and head.

Instantly you are transported back into your room and chair. Feel the weight on your shoulders and your feet grounding you. Sense your spirit fully back and present in your body. Take some really deep breaths again; in through your mouth and out through your mouth into the lower abdomen. Now take two or three in through your nose and out through your mouth. Feel yourself in your chair now.

Grounding/Anchoring Yourself and Golden Bubble of Protection

Sense golden roots coming out of your feet and grounding you on the most beautiful earth. Feel it. Sense a golden bubble all around your aura; it is like extra skin—a layer of protection. It is strong and pliable but impenetrable. Feel it. This golden bubble will be activated indefinitely to protect your energy from negative people or anything environmental. Smile. Take a moment just to say thank you to your body. Your heart, your mind, your soul. Finally, open your eyes whenever you feel ready.

Review

Feel renewed; feel at peace, present and joyful. Expanded in the whole of the heart and chest area. Take notes in your diary—you can read back and reflect on it all when you need to. If you are meditating in a group then allow each person the opportunity to share what magic they have experienced, remembering all the good moments. What did you feel, see, sense, or just know? What lessons can you take away from this that will help you in any way with your beautiful life journey? Feel touched by your beautiful Sacred Heart. Blessed. Smile.

I have been avidly focused on heart-related consciousness for nearly twenty years now my friend. I know there is a movement that highlights scientific research about the congruence of the heart. It is called Heart-Math Solutions. I have been so touched by how this organisation and the spiritual pioneers, of which I hope I am one, are marrying the two camps in a coherent resonance with one another. It is such a joy to see. Remember the ancient Egyptians weight the heart in the underworld to see what sort of person you were in life and Jesus and Mary are always depicted with the sacred Heart emblazoned in their chest.

It really is time to come out of the head and into the heart and allow the heart to teach and lead the way like never before. N.B. Check out Heart Math Solutions book by Doc Children.

Chapter Twenty-Two
Garden of Eden

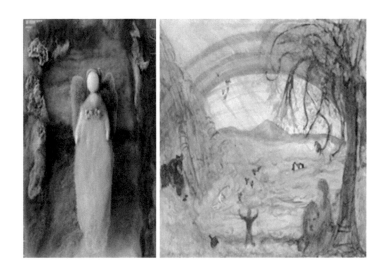

Artwork by Joslin Lambert (left) and Carol Watson (right)

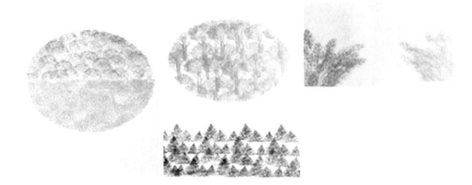

Artwork by Felicity Clyne

[Begin first with your routine.]

Visualise where you live now, and if you will see its boundaries. Sense the sprawl of human activity and the vehicles, animals, trees, buildings and sacred chapels and holy sites. Is there a river or hill in your area? Visualise that in your mind, too. Now begin to see this conscious loving light from Mother Father God or Great Spirit, flush down in waves of love as powerful radiant pearlescent light—light-filled with the rainbow hue and sacred sounds of the spheres. See it anchor in the centre of your community, village, town or city.

See it grounding into the Heart or underbelly of this place. Then deeper into the living matrix of light and the waterways underground. See streams of light streak throughout the underworld. Sense a pulse of pure conscious love from the heart of Gaia or the new Lady Paradisia now, as Heaven and New Earth meet and merge in your home area. Feel this light amplifying and expanding and becoming more intense, as it spreads out like a haze, a wave.

See it. Pour your light from your heart, on a puff into it. (Puff). Add your essence to this powerful activation. See the green areas re-energised and see fruit trees, birds and animals return to these areas. Visualise the aura of the hills or mountains in your region. See the chapel, Temple, historic landmarks and holy sites become filled with light. Watch the dense or grey areas soak up the light and change and glow.

Observe the spiral, the tornado of light from Lady Paradisia ascend and expand even more into the area, the landscape and your region, and then country, as Great Spirits spiral does the same. Look at the natural spots—the streams and rivers and how beautiful and sparkling they are now as well as the parklands. See the trees as beacons of light—cathedrals towering high. Can you see them? See their roots of pure light, penetrating deep.

I'll leave you a couple of minutes now to manifest what you want to see in your community. What you want to enjoy that would be for the greater good of all. Have fun doing it. Make it special. Make it count. Enjoy.

Add now an open, communal community amphitheatre to the parkland, see yourself there with your loved ones, family and friends. Sense music coming alive and see colours dance to the sounds. Taste the colours of the sounds. How magnificent is this? See fireworks explode in front of you all and sense your heart really expand. Archangel Chamuel, the beautiful angel of love and peace descends and bathes you all in pink light.

Your heart opens and flutters, as you receive her love and grace, can you feel it? She lets go of many twin flame doves of peace. Reigniting love's long-forgotten promise to everyone, everywhere. Send a puff of love to her from your heart. Heart to heart connect. Feel it!

Time to give thanks once again to God and to Lady Paradisia and Chamuel. Time to bring yourself back into your body and sacred space. Knowing that you can continue to manifest greater things for yourself and your life by devoting time to do this meditation. Knowing that your life will transform right in front of your eyes (that's a promise) because you know that thought creates reality. Take some nice deep happy breaths.

Bringing Yourself Back into Your Physical Body

It's time to return. See the physical you, standing there, arms wide open welcoming you back with a big smile. Walk towards your physical self and go around the back of you. Step into your physical body one leg at a time, like a hand slipping back into a glove. One arm, then your other arm. Bring your torso back into the body and head.

Instantly you are transported back into your room and chair. Feel the weight on your shoulders and your feet grounding you. Sense your spirit fully back and present in your body. Take some really deep breaths again; in through your mouth and out through your mouth into the lower abdomen. Now take two or three in through your nose and out through your mouth. Feel yourself in your chair now.

Grounding/Anchoring Yourself and Golden Bubble of Protection

Sense golden roots coming out of your feet and grounding you on the most beautiful earth. Feel it. Sense a golden bubble all around your aura; it is like extra skin—a layer of protection. It is strong and pliable but impenetrable. Feel it. This golden bubble will be activated indefinitely to protect your energy from negative people or anything environmental. Smile. Take a moment just to say thank you to your body. Your heart, your mind, your soul. Finally, open your eyes whenever you feel ready.

Review

Feel renewed; feel at peace, present and joyful. Take notes in your diary—you can read back and reflect on it all when you need to. If you are meditating in a group then allow each person the opportunity to share what magic they have experienced, remembering all the good moments. What did you feel, see, sense, or just know? What lessons can you take away from this that will help you in any way with your beautiful life journey? Feel touched and blessed. Smile.

Chapter Twenty-Three
St Germain and the Violet
Cave at Lake Tahoe

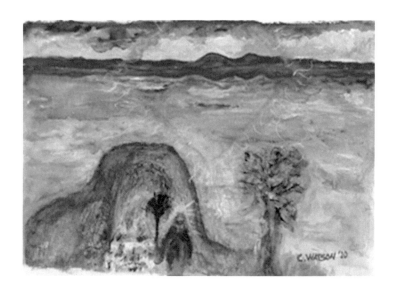

St. Germain or Count of St Germain (1710 – 1784), is a legendary spiritual figure; a master of the ancient arts. He was known for his incredible theosophical and post theosophical knowledge and teachings. He spoke many languages and was known as having had many incarnations. It is thought that St Germain is the catalyst for the New Age Spiritual culture of the Age of Aquarius. He was known as an inventor, alchemist, courtier, adventurer, pianist and amateur composer. Some spiritual thinkers believe he was William Shakespeare (1585 – 1616), in an earlier incarnation.

St. Germain appeared to Guy Ballard, known as the author Godfre Ray King, in 1930 and gave the initial teachings to him whilst channelling this information. "The use of the violet consuming flame is more valuable to you and to all mankind than all the wealth, all the gold and all the jewels of this planet." (The voice of the I AM, January 1941, p. 20). More information is within the books 'Unveiled Mysteries', 'The Magic Presence', and 'the I AM Discourses', Saint Germain.

St Germain Foundation is based in Schaumburg, Illinois, Chicago, USA and in Dunsmuir, California that has been going for around eighty-five years.

Lake Tahoe is a very special node in the Earth's energetic field and you are going to travel to this cave entrance at one of the deepest and purest bodies of water on this beloved planet, which is in North America. It is spiritually known as the inverted (downwards pointing), the pyramid of amethyst energy. (Amethyst is a purple crystal and incredible for its healing properties and also enabling you to connect with the mind's eye, or the third eye easier). Shall we begin?

[Follow your routine.]

As you step out of yourself, you step onto an earthen track in North America that leads towards Lake Tahoe. You see high mountain peaks as you wander toward the lake. You sense and feel a deep connection to this lake and its mysterious depths. You smile as you walk, absorbing the gem energy of the lake itself. Breathing in this ancient place, sensing the Native American Indian energy all around you, sigh from the heart and smile.

Know that this is a very sacred, mystical and magical area and what you are about to experience must be met with your heart open and a sense of wonder and gratitude. You see glimmers of gold and silver dust particles in the air blowing towards you from the Lake. Absorb it all into you, this is magical energy. Remember, you have your special elixir of the New Earth spray in one pocket and a love heart crystal in the other as a gift you will throw into the lake.

You see a deep cave ahead. It's connected to the lake, and it is emitting a sparkling purple light; violet rays pour from the cave and almost wrap around you, welcoming you in. On you go. The air feels more crystalline as you are lured into this incredible cave entrance. Feel the essence of the lake, knowing we are 70% water. Consider how this purest of lakes is effecting our body and the elements inside us, especially the liquid parts of us. Soak it all in. Enjoy.

At the cave entrance, you see a very special master, it is St Germain of the Violet Flame. He lived on this planet in the past and is a Guardian of this

Violet light and essence. Go to him and bow with a big smile. He holds the Violet Flame in his hand, known as the Flame of Transmutation. Walk with him into the peaks and pools of amethyst and violet crystal energy and enjoy.

As you walk now deeper into the interior of the cave corridor, you sense the lake enfolding you in its arms. You are walking under the Lake itself now. You sense the inverted pyramid energy as if there is a funnel pouring down into the core of the earth from here. See an upright pyramid resting over the entire lake and its mirror image upside down, also pointing deep into the heart of the planet.

Can you feel it? You are asked to sit at the very vortex point in the middle of the lake, under the apex of the pyramid above. Breathe and feel the pure essence of this living entity of crystalline water; you may communicate with her spirit. You will experience the living consciousness of Lake Tahoe, as indigenous North Americans would have done for centuries. Feel a flushing and healing filter of light through you, soaking into your cells themselves. How good do you feel?

St Germain summons you to go just a bit further now, to a central area in the cave. There you see an Amethyst purple plinth stone pulsing with violet flames up and through into the air. This is your final initiation. When you stand on the plinth, you allow your body and cells, your aura, all of your being to be cleansed inside and out of all debris and old stuck energy. In those heavenly flames, you will feel renewed. Go ahead, step up on the plinth and feel the violet flames woosh up your body and how good it feels?

It's time to step down and bow and thank St Germain. Ask if you can spray him and the plinth and this lake energy with your New Earth spray now. Give him the gift also—he will know what to do with it. St Germain ushers you back along the corridor and out the cave now. You feel so much gratitude and joy as you say your sincere farewells to St Germain.

It's time to return. See the physical you, standing there, arms wide open welcoming you back with a big smile. Walk towards your physical self and go around the back of you. Step into your physical body one leg at a time, like a glove slipping back in. One arm, then your other arm. Bring your torso back into the body and head.

Instantly you are transported back and into your room and chair. Feel the weight on your shoulders and feet grounding you. Sense your spirit fully back present in your body. Take some really deep breaths again through your mouth and out through your mouth into the lower abdomen. Now two or three in through your nose and out through your mouth now. Feel yourself in your chair now.

Bringing Yourself Back into Your Physical Body

It's time to return. See the physical you, standing there, arms wide open welcoming you back with a big smile. Walk towards your physical self and go around the back of you. Step into your physical body one leg at a time, like a hand slipping back into a glove. One arm, then your other arm. Bring your torso back into the body and head.

Instantly you are transported back into your room and chair. Feel the weight on your shoulders and your feet grounding you. Sense your spirit fully back and present in your body. Take some really deep breaths again; in through your mouth and out through your mouth into the lower abdomen. Now take two or three in through your nose and out through your mouth. Feel yourself in your chair now.

Grounding/Anchoring Yourself and Golden Bubble of Protection

Sense golden roots coming out of your feet and grounding you on the most beautiful earth. Feel it. Sense a golden bubble all around your aura; it is like extra skin—a layer of protection. It is strong and pliable but impenetrable. Feel it. This golden bubble will be activated indefinitely to protect your energy from negative people or anything environmental. Smile. Take a moment just to say thank you to your body. Your heart, your mind, your soul. Finally, open your eyes whenever you feel ready.

Review

Feel renewed; feel at peace, present and joyful. Take notes in your diary—you can read back and reflect on it all when you need to. If you are meditating in a group then allow each person the opportunity to share what magic they have experienced, remembering all the good moments. What did you feel, see, sense, or just know? What lessons can you take away from this that will help you in any way with your beautiful life journey? Feel touched and blessed. Smile.

Chapter Twenty-Four
Stairway in the Clouds

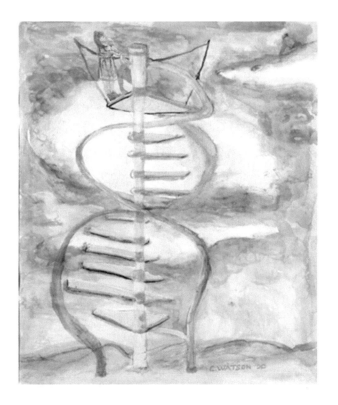

"It's hard to be clear about who you are when you are carrying around a bunch of baggage from the past. I've learned to let go and move more quickly into the next place."

– Angelina Jolie

The purpose of this meditation is to assist you in surrendering all that you carry on your back and shoulders, relieving the burden of the past that sometimes can weigh so heavy.

[Full routine first.]

I want you to sense the most divine golden sun, way up in the Galaxy. I want you to imagine taking your mind way up there to bask in that incredible light.

You see a marble-white shining stairway up in the clouds, with a smooth white rail at one side of the wide steps—this is your stairway in the clouds. How gorgeous does it look as it peeks out from the cloud above, with all that incredible sunlight; ancient golden sunlight bathing it, cradling it in the love of that pure light. Feel yourself raised up and into that amazing cloud way up above, where the sun is filtering all that golden-white rays down and onto the cloud surface.

In an instant, you are way up there. How does it feel? What do you sense and see? The perspective is totally different from up here. How do you look? Look down at your feet and see what is on them and what you are wearing.

Feel the presence of Divine Spirit, Great Spirit's essence and immense love bathing you, soaking and saturating into you. Grab hold of the handrail and, feeling truly supported, step onto the first step downwards.

You are going to call up anything you wish you acknowledge that has been a niggle, a gripe, or a challenge of late that has annoyed or upset you. On that first step, you let it really come up into your awareness. Feel it. It's safe to do this. When you take that next step down you release it as the marble soaks it up.

Take the step... how good does that feel? Say thank you to that feeling or thought that you had, and for all, it taught you. We are here to experience, and this is just another one of those experiences. We can choose to repeat these feelings or thoughts, or just acknowledge them and move on to the next, more positive feeling.

Every thought or feeling is a teacher. We can repeat ground-hog day, or learn and grow from it, recognising our patterns and how we behave with these thoughts and feelings. We all want to evolve and this experience is just a teacher for you, so thank it. Feels good right? Feel it, as it literally soaks out of you into the marble step; as if you are a sponge letting go of excess.

Now call up anything deeper, ongoing issues, something you never talk about but that really does affect you on a regular basis that might be left unexpressed. Call it up; it is safe to do so. Thank this issue for all it has taught you about experiencing that particular emotion. How good does it feel to get rid of it? It leaves more space for good thoughts and feelings, right?

Continue down your marble staircase, calling up and releasing all those outdated, old, negative thoughts and feelings. Remember you are more than that. You never get it wrong; we are all perfect in all our imperfections. Your loved ones are all perfect in their imperfections too. Keep going down, feel the warm wind in your face and through your clothes.

It feels amazing. Even your feet feel happy, yes—happy feet with the warm air around them. Smile. Give thanks to the Great Spirit above and within you. Thank the beautiful new earth we live in. Gratitude is the thing that brings more good to us when we just stop and say thank you to things or people we interact with every day.

As you get closer to the ground you feel that so much baggage and weight really has lifted off your shoulders. You have a lights-on-moment, or an epiphany that all that rubbish was just that that you have continuously carried about like a sack of potatoes on your back. You feel more space in your mind, right? There is a lightness in and around you; in fact, you sense you are more a part of the light all around and through you. You feel more connected.

How good does that feel? You feel there is now more room for positive thoughts. More lightness in your body too, which will give you a lot more energy. Feel how happy your organs are and smile. Say thank you. We never acknowledge our internal landscape, our organs, heart, mind, soul, our bones, our cells.

Say 'thank you', and smile as you reach the ground. Sigh a big sigh of relief. How good was that? Amazing right? Time to return to your physical, beautiful, happy body. Do this exercise as often as you need it. Let this beautiful meditation work for you. Share it with others who may need it. Help those that need a hand when they are struggling. This will lighten their load too.

Bringing Yourself Back into Your Physical Body

It's time to return. See the physical you, standing there, arms wide open welcoming you back with a big smile. Walk towards your physical self and go around the back of you. Step into your physical body one leg at a time, like a hand slipping back into a glove. One arm, then your other arm. Bring your torso back into the body and head.

Instantly you are transported back into your room and chair. Feel the weight on your shoulders and your feet grounding you. Sense your spirit fully back and present in your body. Take some really deep breaths again; in through your mouth and out through your mouth into the lower abdomen. Now take two or three in through your nose and out through your mouth. Feel yourself in your chair now.

Grounding/Anchoring Yourself and Golden Bubble of Protection

Sense golden roots coming out of your feet and grounding you on the most beautiful earth. Feel it. Sense a golden bubble all around your aura; it is like extra skin—a layer of protection. It is strong and pliable but impenetrable. Feel it. This golden bubble will be activated indefinitely to protect your energy from negative people or anything environmental. Smile. Take a moment just to say thank you to your body. Your heart, your mind, your soul. Finally, open your eyes whenever you feel ready.

Review

Feel renewed; feel at peace, present and joyful. Take notes in your diary—you can read back and reflect on it all when you need to. If you are meditating in a group then allow each person the opportunity to share what magic they have experienced, remembering all the good moments. What did you feel, see, sense, or just know? What lessons can you take away from this that will help you in any way with your beautiful life journey? Feel touched and blessed. Smile.

Chapter Twenty-Five
Casting the Net

This is a meditation all about manifesting your abundance and enhancing personal virtues. It is an empowering one; one that allows you to project what you want things to be like in your future.

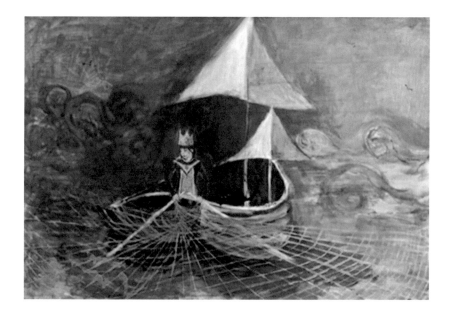

Painting by Ele Alba

[Refer to Chapter Two for the full Routine that includes the Breathwork and Pillar of Light Anchoring.]

As you step out of your physical body and into your light body, you see in front of you a stone wall hugging a tiny cute wee harbour. In the harbour is your own personal boat. You see it in the low water, as the tide is getting ready to gently come into the harbour and launch your boat. There are stone steps leading down into it. It is a twenty-eight foot, beautiful boat.

It is motorised and has a very comfortable big chair with a blanket and cushions by a golden fishing net—your net. On you go. Head for the harbour wall and take the steps down into the boat. The rope will be released when you are on board and ready to take off. Step onboard and settle down; get rugged up for this short trip out into the open ocean.

You are safe. The engine fires up, you don't need to do anything whatsoever; just relax and enjoy the sights. Take in the sounds of the noisy seagulls, listen to the splash of the water, smell the salt air. Feel the breeze on your skin. The boat fires up and takes off, slowly manoeuvring out of the tiny harbour.

Smile and feel excited about this adventure ahead. Consider it a Manifestation journey. Feel the waves as your small vessel gently bobs up and down as it heads from the harbour and slowly leaves the shore. This scene can be anywhere you want it to be—any coastline that comes to your mind. Look back and admire it as you go further and further out into open water.

You feel so held, so safe; everything is effortless and easy and joyous. The seagulls are still flying overhead, squawking away. Watch them and their antics. They dive-bomb into the ocean and play tag with one another. It's magical to watch. You feel so much part of this great conscious expanse. Feel the depth of the ocean and the depth of your own unconscious mind. You see the beautiful sparkling golden net close by. This net reflects your consciousness and sub-consciousness. It is your manifestation net.

Lie back on your lounging chair, cosy up. Shut your eyes and think of the personal virtues you have, and how you can harness these and make them even more alive in you to create the most harmonious loving relationships on a multitude of levels. These levels incorporate such things as patience, tolerance, forgiveness, gratitude, open honesty, clarity about your feelings, etc. Think about each important personal relationship now and how it operates, how it works or doesn't work so well and what virtues would enhance it.

Take time now to go within, deep into the living memory field, the consciousness; look for patterns; good ones and bad ones. Was there any snowball effect happening from yourself that made things spiral downwards and found wings to affect other areas of your relationship and life? Be honest and vulnerable with yourself and seek gentle, inner truth.

Consider the virtues of honesty would really help make each relationship better. Do this by thinking of people you really truly admire by their great virtues—consider how they act or react to things. Sense a drawing of these to you.

It's time, the golden net will need cast overboard now. So, rise and grab hold of it, feel it in your fingers as you stretch to the side with it in your hands and throw it out over the boat ridge, into the deep blue water. You hear it splice through the water; listen to the sound of it and watch it sink into the deep. It will get hauled as the motor starts up and gently trawls for these virtues for you in your own depths of feeling. Feel the net in your hands getting filled up with them. How great does that feel? See these virtues as golden nuggets, instead of fish; lightweight golden nuggets.

The boat slows and stops to let you easily and gently draw up your net full of the virtues you have harnessed. Bring the net up and back on board. You see the nuggets and as you bring the net right on board you feel them fizz and filter like golden stardust into your body. Feel it. How great is that? Smile.

Now it's time to go deep again; settle back in your cosy chair with the blanket. Contemplate what are your true heart desires, what do you want in your life right now, what traits do you want to be remembered by? Not only in your personal life but creative or work life? Really go deep. How do you see things?

If you go five years ahead, what does it look like, this rewarding, satisfying and fulfilling life? See it in multi-colour; large and bright and full of sound, full of life and energy. See and feel it. When you are ready rise again and cast out your net to harness this life from your deep subconscious mind, as represented by the deep ocean of potential. Haul it on board now and again feel all this potential sprinkle into you as your net is drawn on board.

Feel it—all those goals, dreams and heart's desires you have about your relationships. Think about your old relationships, your new ones, those with family, friends and loved ones, all coming back alive and illuminated. Manifest more positive feelings about going forward in your life, renewed with work and also creative ideas. Feel yourself renewed, with a refreshed sense of how you can fulfil your life and feel satisfied. Feels good right?

It's time to head back for shore as the boat gently turns from the deep ocean of your own consciousness, for the shallow shores of your life. See the horizon and the land with its hills and buildings, the harbour. See yourself at the harbour waving you back, ready to anchor your rope to the round iron bollard. Ready to welcome you home to your physical self. Smile as you throw the large rope up to your physical self and step off the boat now.

Bringing Yourself Back into Your Physical Body

It's time to return. See the physical you, standing there, arms wide open welcoming you back with a big smile. Walk towards your physical self and go around the back of you. Step into your physical body one leg at a time, like a hand slipping back into a glove. One arm, then your other arm. Bring your torso back into the body and head.

Instantly you are transported back into your room and chair. Feel the weight on your shoulders and your feet grounding you. Sense your spirit fully back and present in your body. Take some really deep breaths again; in through your mouth and out through your mouth into the lower abdomen. Now take two or three in through your nose and out through your mouth. Feel yourself in your chair now.

Grounding/Anchoring Yourself and Golden Bubble of Protection

Sense golden roots coming out of your feet and grounding you on the most beautiful earth. Feel it. Sense a golden bubble all around your aura; it is like extra skin—a layer of protection. It is strong and pliable but impenetrable. Feel it. This golden bubble will be activated indefinitely to protect your energy from negative people or anything environmental. Smile. Take a moment just to say thank you to your body. Your heart, your mind, your soul. Finally, open your eyes whenever you feel ready.

Review

How wonderful to focus on personal manifestation again. I hope you benefit from doing this one regularly. Add in your Affirmations to enhance and power up your work.

Feel renewed; feel at peace, present and joyful. Take notes in your diary—you can read back and reflect on it all when you need to. If you are meditating in a group then allow each person the opportunity to share what magic they have experienced, remembering all the good moments. What did you feel, see, sense, or just know? What lessons can you take away from this that will help you in any way with your beautiful life journey? Feel touched and blessed. Smile.

Chapter Twenty-Six
Hawk's Nest

This is a truly magical experience and allows you the opportunity to have a 'bird's-eye view'—quite literally and psychically of being a Hawk's chick. This will help you to really connect with the two-legged kingdom and be bestowed with wisdom from this Hawk Mother.

The Hawk is thought of as a Solar Bird. In the past, Druids would dress in bird or hawk feathers, to perform rituals in ancient times in Scotland. You will meet the hawk way up high; either upon a cliff ledge or a tall tree near the top of the forest canopy. The choice will be yours as you become a chick in her nest. It will be an immersive experience, as you fully become part of her care in the safety of her habitat.

– Adapted from the *Druid Animal Oracle* book by Philip and
Stephanie Carr-Gomm

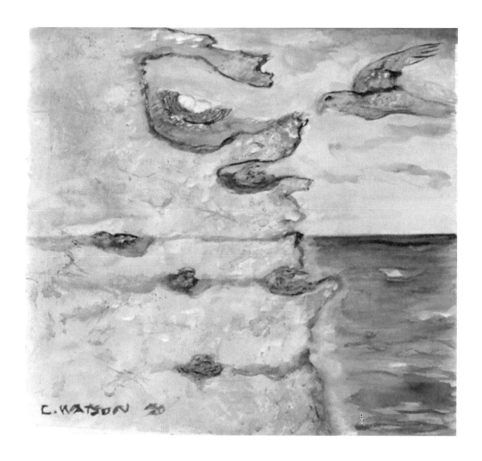

C.WATSON 20

[As always, do remember to begin with the full routine.]

Firstly, feel yourself shrink but also rise at the same time. It is easy and effortless as you are caught up in the warm thermals of the land. You can see cliffs and ocean ahead and on top of the cliffs, you spot a forest. Choose where you wish to experience this incredible journey and head for it. If it is the cliff edge, you will see a grassy ledge jutting out high up on the grey cliff face.

You see the whole rock face dotted by washes of white bird droppings and hear a variety of birds as you head for your nest. If it is in the tree canopy close to the cliff you will see the large nest snug in between two very large branches. From that tree, there is a very large gap in the woods so you can see quite a distance from it.

The Hawk is expecting you and you can sense her majestic colours and feathers; the yellow beak and big round, black eyes. Can you see her as you land comfortably in the nest? Feel her off in the distance and send her love and gratitude for this connection and for all she is going to share with you.

Now, look around your nest. The intricacy of the home is amazing. Hundreds of tiny little willow twigs, tiny twigs and down from other trees and bushes. Feel how comfortable and safe you are; so high up, like a wee bird in her magnificent nest. Her home feels warm and comfortable and the outlook is fantastic—so high up. The Hawk teaches you to see from a higher perspective and an understanding of how it feels to be one of the Queens or Kings of the skies. She will remind you that you can also be hawk-eyed as you observe all around you. What do you see?

The hawk helps you understand how to assemble missing pieces of your life's framework. Seeing three hundred and sixty degrees in all directions and from above, as you connect with the golden light of the sun. This is the inspiration solar energy can offer you. You can feel your nest bathed in sunlight.

The hawk has also been connected to human beings for many years, as she has been linked to nobility especially during medieval times as they were used for sport as Kings and Queens held the hawk in his or her leather glove. The hawk is noble and connected to chivalry too. Feel the presence of this beautiful and striking bird.

Call out to her to come to you in your nest and see what she does. This is your time to connect with her and speak to her about any issues you feel she could enlighten you with. Enjoy the experience and your time with her.

How was that? Now she wants to teach you to fly, to conquer your fear and see things from a much higher perspective. Go fly with her. How does that feel?

Friends, it's time to say your thanks and goodbyes. It's time to fly for home now, catching the warm thermals as you go. Hawk takes off in all her majesty and heads back for her nest.

What will you remember from this experience, what have you learnt that you can take with you and integrate into your own life?

You descend now over the land and see the physical you there on the horizon.

Bringing Yourself Back into Your Physical Body

It's time to return. See the physical you, standing there, arms wide open welcoming you back with a big smile. Walk towards your physical self and go around the back of you. Step into your physical body one leg at a time, like a hand slipping back into a glove. One arm, then your other arm. Bring your torso back into the body and head.

Instantly you are transported back into your room and chair. Feel the weight on your shoulders and your feet grounding you. Sense your spirit fully back and present in your body. Take some really deep breaths again; in through your mouth and out through your mouth into the lower abdomen. Now take two or three in through your nose and out through your mouth. Feel yourself in your chair now.

Grounding/Anchoring Yourself and Golden Bubble of Protection

Sense golden roots coming out of your feet and grounding you on the most beautiful earth. Feel it. Sense a golden bubble all around your aura; it is like extra skin—a layer of protection. It is strong and pliable but impenetrable. Feel it. This golden bubble will be activated indefinitely to protect your energy from negative people or anything environmental. Smile. Take a moment just to say thank you to your body. Your heart, your mind, your soul. Finally, open your eyes whenever you feel ready.

Review

Feel renewed; feel at peace, present and joyful. Take notes in your diary—you can read back and reflect on it all when you need to. If you are meditating in a group then allow each person the opportunity to share what magic they have experienced, remembering all the good moments. What did you feel, see, sense, or just know? What lessons can you take away from this that will help you in any way with your beautiful life journey? Feel touched and blessed.

I feel humbled and little when I do this meditation. I really feel I am the chick in the Hawks nest and I am reliant on her to provide for me. It allows me a deep resonance with this creature. Respect and a love for the two-legged teachers of this world. I hope it does for you too.

Smile.

Chapter Twenty-Seven
Meeting St Brigid and
Goddess Ceridwen at the
Standing Stone Circle

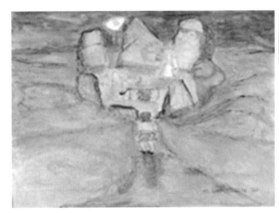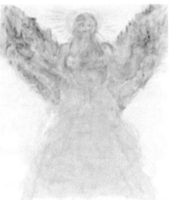

Artwork by Carol Watson

Both of these Deities are from the Irish Tradition. This meditation is an adaptation from the Author Cairistiona Worthington's Oracle Cards and Book, 'A Beginners Guide to Druids' the book is summed up in its header, 'The Guardians of Alchemical Transformation. The Alchemy of Healing'. This meditation focuses on looking within and working with your body's elemental nature in a stone circle set in Ireland.

Stepping out of your skin in your translucent body, you are transported to a wild and natural place, a valley in Kildare, Southern Ireland, to St Brigid's holy well for a blessing, before walking to her standing stone circle to meet her and Ceridwen. You can feel the energy of this Emerald Isle envelope you and welcome your spirit here. You see the circular stone well in front of you with a small bucket and scoop spoon hanging from it. Take the spoon and dip it into the holy well. Drink the water and bless yourself with it also. Ask St Brigid to please come and meet you and take you into the standing stone circle for this ceremonial healing and to meet Goddess Ceridwen. The earthy, Celtic, Irish Mother. The Goddess. On you go and enjoy. Remember to bow to St Brigid when you meet, knowing you have the New Earth elixir spray in your pocket and two love heart crystal thank-you gifts in the other. On you go and meet her.

Together you walk into the standing stone circle and see a cauldron pot on a metal rod over an unlit fire pit. She leaves you to go in yourself to observe the cauldron pot. It is very important you look at its structure, colour, texture, thickness and its age. Every minute detail is important to notice before we begin. Has it any cracks, is it well used? Has it a thin or thick rim; is it small, or is this cauldron pot large and wide open? How do you feel about it? It is your cauldron pot.

As you stand beside it, St Brigid enters the circle with a golden ladle in hand, which she will use later. She welcomes this enormous light into the circle as you watch Goddess Ceridwen descend from the heavens and land beside St Brigid. Observe how awesome she looks as she begins to take form. Notice her hair, eyes, her clothing and do the same with St Brigid.

Notice everything. How do they feel to you? Bow and smile to them both, feel your heart rise, open and expand to them. Send a puff of love to them both now. Both of them smile at you with their mouths and eyes. Feel their heart radiating love out to you and the stones around them. Feel the presence of the stones. You realise this truly is a sacred ritual circle and you are about to be part of it. It is in your honour.

St. Brigid hands you a lighter and asks you to light your cauldron fire with the twigs and sticks underneath it. When you do you can sense the earth beneath your feet and how it holds the fire and the pot in its arms. Feel the air element, the wind around you. Observe how the fire looks. Is it being blown by the wind up one side of the pot, is it a simmering flame or a huge burning flame under the centre of the pot, look at how the wind and the flames react and how the cauldron pot receives the flame.

Now go and take a look inside the pot at the liquid in it. Is it simmering underneath and flat on top, or is it bubbling over? What is the colour of the liquid, and what is its consistency? How do you think it would taste?

St Brigid steps close now with her golden ladle and offers you her golden elixir. As she holds it to your lips, you sup it and feel its energy; it is healing energy and very potent. Feel the warmth or coolness of it, feel where it goes to in your body from your mouth. Is there any area that needs this healing, or some attention? Feel it. Is it a clouded head, a negative mind you have? A constricted throat, or agitated stomach?

The Mother Goddess beckons you over now to talk to her, one-to-one, about any issue troubling you. This is your time and you can give her the gift and holy blessing at the end of your chat. Enjoy. Speak from your heart. Do it now. Make it count.

Give your thanks for her counsel and bow with a beautiful, wide smile. Go to St Brigid and offer her your gift and a blessing with the New Earth holy water too. She receives it with gratitude and bows, smiling at you.

Feel the power of this ritual and the energy of the standing stones too. The living stones. Go and spray each of them as a blessing.

It's time to say goodbye and leave these two remarkable Goddesses. Leaving the circle, you wave and smile.

Bringing Yourself Back into Your Physical Body

It's time to return. See the physical you, standing there, arms wide open welcoming you back with a big smile. Walk towards your physical self and go around the back of you. Step into your physical body one leg at a time, like a hand slipping back into a glove. One arm, then your other arm. Bring your torso back into the body and head.

Instantly you are transported back into your room and chair. Feel the weight on your shoulders and your feet grounding you. Sense your spirit fully back and present in your body. Take some really deep breaths again; in through your mouth and out through your mouth into the lower abdomen. Now take two or three in through your nose and out through your mouth. Feel yourself in your chair now.

Grounding/Anchoring Yourself and Golden Bubble of Protection

Sense golden roots coming out of your feet and grounding you on the most beautiful earth. Feel it. Sense a golden bubble all around your aura; it is like extra skin—a layer of protection. It is strong and pliable but impenetrable. Feel it. This golden bubble will be activated indefinitely to protect your energy from negative people or anything environmental. Smile. Take a moment just to say thank you to your body. Your heart, your mind, your soul. Finally, open your eyes whenever you feel ready.

Review

Feel renewed; feel at peace, present and joyful. Take notes in your diary—you can read back and reflect on it all when you need to. If you are meditating in a group then allow each person the opportunity to share what magic they have experienced, remembering all the good moments. What did you feel, see, sense, or just know? What lessons can you take away from this that will help you in any way with your beautiful life journey? Feel touched and blessed. Smile.

In your notes, Please spend some extra time considering how your cauldron pot looked like as this represents you and your physicality; your body. Is it worn out, or shiny and robust. How was the brew, this represents your emotional life—was it calm and tasty or bubbling over? How was the fire element that represents your passions, drive, energy levels? Was it too strong in your left feminine side or was there not enough flame energy? Think of the wind as representing your mental faculties; was your thinking focused and not too all over the place' was it guiding the fire, or were you?

Chapter Twenty-Eight
The Horse Whisperer

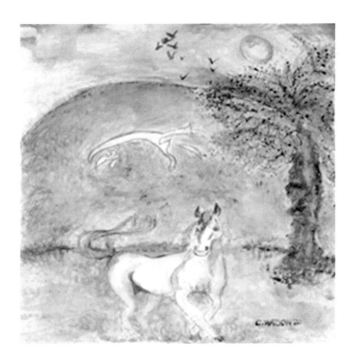

[Begin with your routine.]

The horse, in the Celtic tradition, represents the fecundity of the land and life. The horse is full of sensual sexuality too. In the past, kings were married to white horses, in a symbolic fashion in Ireland. The symbolism linked both horse and King in a powerful sovereign bond. Uffington, Oxfordshire in England has huge chalk marking in the hillside depicting how important the essence and energy of the sacred horse was. She is linked to the energy of the Dragon and all the virtues of the spirit of the dragon. This gorgeous meditation will bring

you so close to the spirit of the white horse mother, allowing you to take on her
powerful characteristics.

See the white horse on the hill, where you will bless her with the new earth elixir. Leave the gift for the dragon at the foot of the hill, in a cluster of stones. Remember to Bless that spot also. Firstly, though, look at the beauty of this amazing ancient chalk etching. Send her love from your heart. Ask her to communicate with you.

Think of the forms of horse that have inspired humanity; such as the Kelpies in the Scottish tradition, and Rhiannon or Epony in Irish and Welsh lore. Or perhaps you connect your imagination more intensely with the mystical Unicorn or Pegasus horse Goddesses? Feel your heart connect and open to see what the white horse shows you. How magnificent was that? Speak to her about anything troubling you in the present or from your past. She has the power to take you to read your Akashic Records, where you may read the imprint of energy from your past and old pasts.

Rise now. Go climb the hillside and leave your offering and bless her. Feel the steepness as you go tentatively up the grassy hill. How was that? Now bless her. How does it feel being in the presence of this carving into the land, knowing it is thousands of years old? You feel part of the hill and her, right? In awe.

Ok, as you look below into your meadow you see a magnificent white horse. What aspects of her do you notice in particular? She is waiting for you. You are going to go on a ride around the field with her, or maybe further. Maybe she'll take you into the sky. You will be able to absorb her light and love and feel it imbued into your own muscles as you both become one.

On you go. You reach the ground and first bless the dragon with your elixir and love heart gift. Smile and feel the dragon spirit smile back at you. Look at your white charger, she is galloping right over the meadow towards you. Watch. Observe everything.

How does she look and feel? Feel her majesty and sheer power. She stops and bows her head to you as you do back. What aspect is she showing you? She may show you something in her actions that is a message for you now about your life. Look carefully. Ask her if you are unclear about the meaning. Thank her.

On you go. Touch her, brush and stroke her with your hands. Feel the muscles twitch. She is so sensitive. Ask if she will take you on a ride. If she agrees you will know. This is your time, enjoy. Make it count. Make this a truly memorable experience. Invite your inner child and inner aspects to be with you, to rise in you so all parts of you get to enjoy this experience. On you go.

She slows down and comes to a stop by the gate. It's time to get off and thank her. You have one more hidden gift of a long necklace, with another love heart on the pendant. Put it over her neck. Say thank you and bow with a smile of reverence and love.

It's time to return. You turn around and see your physical self.

Bringing Yourself Back into Your Physical Body

It's time to return. See the physical you, standing there, arms wide open welcoming you back with a big smile. Walk towards your physical self and go around the back of you. Step into your physical body one leg at a time, like a hand slipping back into a glove. One arm, then your other arm. Bring your torso back into the body and head.

Instantly you are transported back into your room and chair. Feel the weight on your shoulders and your feet grounding you. Sense your spirit fully back and present in your body. Take some really deep breaths again; in through your mouth and out through your mouth into the lower abdomen. Now take two or three in through your nose and out through your mouth. Feel yourself in your chair now.

Grounding/Anchoring Yourself and Golden Bubble of Protection

Sense golden roots coming out of your feet and grounding you on the most beautiful earth. Feel it. Sense a golden bubble all around your aura; it is like extra skin—a layer of protection. It is strong and pliable but impenetrable. Feel it. This golden bubble will be activated indefinitely to protect your energy from negative people or anything environmental. Smile. Take a moment just to say thank you to your body. Your heart, your mind, your soul. Finally, open your eyes whenever you feel ready.

Review

Feel renewed; feel at peace, present and joyful. Take notes in your diary—you can read back and reflect on it all when you need to. If you are meditating in a group then allow each person the opportunity to share what magic they have experienced, remembering all the good moments. What did you feel, see, sense, or just know? What lessons can you take away from this that will help you in any way with your beautiful life journey? Feel touched and blessed. Smile.

Chapter Twenty-Nine
Year/Life Review

"It is on the strength of observation and reflection that one finds a way. So we must dig and delve unceasingly."

–Claude Monet

Life is a journey and we face many clouds on our personal Rainbow Path. However, friend, it is the life we put into living that really matters and the gratitude for each experience that enlightens and challenges us to stretch and become greater. These are the gifts. So this meditation is all about reviewing where you've been and where you want to go. It allows you that wee bit of time out to just be present and mindful of your past and see what you have learned, in order to walk forward with more clarity and direction. Enjoy.

[Begin with your routine. Light Body]

Step out of your dense physical body now, which is a light-body—a mirror of yourself. I will guide you safely back at the very end of the journey and ground and anchor you safely. I will also Protect your aura. It's safe to journey with me.

You step onto a forested path and ahead of you is a gleaming marble temple. It is small and has steps leading up to the entrance, with pillars at the top on either side. Two large ornate heavy doors begin to open as you walk towards this illuminated structure. It is your auditorium and film-house. On you go, head for it.

As you begin slowly walking up those steps, you feel a flush of starlight pouring out of the mini theatre; your theatre. It feels so inviting and embracing as this light swirls around you and gently draws you towards the doors and into the Temple. You see an ornate red velvet throne with a footstool and nothing else. It's surrounded by white walls and what looks like small circular floor lights all around the base of the walls in this circular space. Go take a seat and settle in. You see a remote control, which you can sit with.

The lights dim as you soon become immersed in blackness now. A full surround cinema screen comes on in front of you; the screen is pearlescent and surrounds you in this tiny wee Temple. A beautiful lady's voice comes through the hidden speakers and asks you to press the green button on the remote control, which will take you back down the timeline to your baby and childhood years. You will see flashes of people, places, scenes, scenarios that in some way might benefit you reviewing from this perspective of the observer.

You will not feel any emotion, as you are only the witness to great things, and difficult things that occurred for you in the distant past. Time to review. You can fast forward, freeze frame and look at the situation from above, the side, from stepping into your skin (or the other person in the scenario's skin) if you need to understand the reason for certain words or actions. This will allow you to see all sides of the story, from every possible angle and see the positive lesson within it.

Take as long as you like; it is your journey. Do make sure though that you understand the positive message and lesson from each situation. When you go back and look at things, you get to reclaim your inner territory and the light of awareness helps heal anything that is stuck in you or is heavy and weighs you down. Old wounds can be healed.

Time to press the 'forward' orange button and leap ahead to childhood, to review all key landmarks both positive and difficult and again see the lessons from it. Now again press the orange button that takes you ahead again into your teenage and adolescent years. Which challenges did you overcome and what learning did you get from this time? Scenes will appear and you may see a variety of people; ones who supported you, ones that challenged you, and those that you helped along the way too and bonded with. What major things need to be faced and healed and what growth did you gain from some of your challenges?

Pressing the orange remote, you come into adulthood and the first job you had and the first really important serious relationship. Look at them and feel into things. How did you handle all these new responsibilities at work and how did you manage? Did you put energy into your work? Were you shy? Did you strive and not be recognised or was it the opposite? How would you have done things differently at all, with all the years of wisdom you have now? Look at your relationships with friends—were they real and meaningful? Were you shallow or deep with them? Include your personal, intimate relationships in these thoughts. What would you change or do differently?

The screen fades now into blackness and a map appears on the screen. It is leading you to roadblocks, crossroads, U-turns you took or still need to take in your current time frame. Have a look at the map and recognise what these key landmarks are about, are they repeating negative patterns at all; if so what are they about? What fears have you carried forward into this now-time? Images will form on the screen to help you understand.

Observe yourself. Look seven hundred and twenty degrees, all around you at the situations, and from different perspectives, also look within yourself at your patterns. Know it is a safe place to do this work, you are only the observer witness.

The lights dim on screen again as you sit a minute and think of a note you could have written to yourself now, when you were, say, seven years old. What advice would you have liked to hear? See the words on the screen pop up now. Take it all in.

Now the screen fades to black again and you see a red racing car come up on the screen side on, it is your wee car, your mode of transport into the future. Imagine yourself stepping into the beautiful car. It is on a fun racing track that goes all the way around the temple walls. How great is this? You are in for a ride now. Buckle up and before you turn the engine ignition on, think of where you are going now in your life, where you want things to be steered with your relationships at home, friendships, close and intimate relationships, in your community and with new connections from course or workshops or groups you want to be part of in the present.

Look at your work and creative life, fun, adventurous plus your spiritual life. What do you want to happen? Make it big. Don't dare hold back, make it beyond your wildest dreams. You have to think about it to manifest these ideas into reality. How does that all feel? Empowering, exciting, fantastic? It can be all these things if you want it to be. You can do this or anything you set your mind to.

Now for the fun bit…fire up your engine and go around the track as fast or cautiously as you want—it's your ride; it will go round and round the circuit. Enjoy.

It's time to bring the car to a stop, as it's time to leave this Temple space and return to your life—hopefully invigorated and brighter, clearer, more assured about yourself. The lights come on and the doors open wide.

Bringing Yourself Back into Your Physical Body

It's time to return. See the physical you, standing there, arms wide open welcoming you back with a big smile. Walk towards your physical self and go around the back of you. Step into your physical body one leg at a time, like a hand slipping back into a glove. One arm, then your other arm. Bring your torso back into the body and head.

Instantly you are transported back into your room and chair. Feel the weight on your shoulders and your feet grounding you. Sense your spirit fully back and present in your body. Take some really deep breaths again; in through your mouth and out through your mouth into the lower abdomen. Now take two or three in through your nose and out through your mouth. Feel yourself in your chair now.

Grounding/Anchoring Yourself and Golden Bubble of Protection

Sense golden roots coming out of your feet and grounding you on the most beautiful earth. Feel it. Sense a golden bubble all around your aura; it is like extra skin—a layer of protection. It is strong and pliable but impenetrable. Feel it. This golden bubble will be activated indefinitely to protect your energy from negative people or anything environmental. Smile. Take a moment just to say thank you to your body. Your heart, your mind, your soul. Finally, open your eyes whenever you feel ready.

Review

Feel renewed; feel at peace, present and joyful. Take notes in your diary—you can read back and reflect on it all when you need to. If you are meditating in a group then allow each person the opportunity to share what magic they have experienced, remembering all the good moments. What did you feel, see, sense, or just know? What lessons can you take away from this that will help you in any way with your beautiful life journey? Feel touched and blessed. Smile.

Chapter Thirty
Stepping Stones

"There will always be rocks in the road ahead of us. They will be stumbling blocks or stepping stones; depending on how you use them."

– Friedrich Nietzsche (1844 – 1900) German Philosopher and Cultural Critic

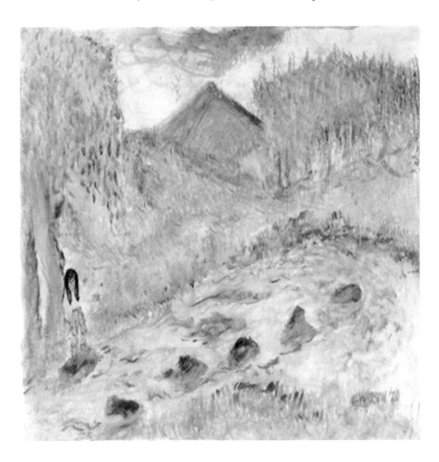

[Begin with your routine. Light Body]

Step out of your dense physical body now, which is a light-body—a mirror of yourself. I will guide you safely back at the very end of the journey and ground and anchor you safely. I will also Protect your aura. It's safe to journey with me.

I would like to guide you on an amazing scenic journey to the Highlands of Scotland, or to a special rugged and rural landscape of your choosing. I will transport you to a beautiful clearing by a forest, with a river running through it. Let's journey—join me.

You see the image right in front of you like a muted, gorgeous watercolour painting. Roll your trousers up and take off your shoes and socks and walk through the luscious green grass, towards a nice tall tree by the banks of your pristine and sparkling blue river. Smell the air, look out for the blackbirds and any other land animal around. If you are in the Highlands, you will see long red-haired Highland cows grazing the land; they are just such magical and primaeval creatures. They can be in your landscape too if you choose.

The sky is dark and blue, it is very atmospheric. The temperature is mild, not too hot, and there is a lovely gentle refreshing breeze sweeping through your hair as you walk to your river.

The closer you get, the clearer your river looks. See those large boulders in the water, they are spaced out perfectly to cross to the other side. These rocks are important landmarks for you. It is a deeply spiritual journey you will go on, as you leap from one boulder to the other.

The first stepping stone you leap onto represents your biggest worry right now if you have any or your biggest challenge. It may represent a health issue, work worries, about a family member or money worries. Or something else. As with everything, the first one is always the hardest to tackle until we commit and get going, taking on the challenges.

On you go think of what your major concern is right now that you're working through. Observe it as a distant spectator and see it from all angles, or dimensions, from all timelines and from the perspective of anyone who may be concerned. When you have looked at all the angles, focus on the positive lesson it has been trying to teach you. Do you get it now? If you feel you have a clearer understanding of it and how you can overcome it and learn from it then go take a leap onto your next boulder, it will be a little wobbly but you will steady yourself when you land and re-balance your footing. Great—how good did that jump feel? Like a leap of faith, right? Feel the gift of having tackled that head-on.

Call forward the next worry you have and again look at it from all angles and what you can learn from it in a positive, constructive way? Will it make you more confident to speak out or hold back if you tackle this one? What is it about and how burdened are you with it?

This one is a little further set out than the last one, but you know you can handle a wobbly stone and you can handle this one too, so on you go and take a leap over to it. It is a wee bit slippery with the slime on the rock but you steady yourself once again and get ready to face the next stepping stone in your life. What is it? Think about it as you face your next rock in the river. Call it up and face this one, as you did with the other two.

You've got this. See it from all angles and all people involved. How can you evolve and grow from this one? It doesn't look like such a big leap to reach this stone; in fact, it is also flat as a pancake so it will be a doddle just to step onto its surface. Go for it. Now finish off the steps as you look at the final three rocks in the river that takes you to new, dry land. Also a new brighter future for you symbolically. The sun's rays are actually bathing the banks of the river on the other side. Go for it. Enjoy.

How much fun was that, as well as a useful exercise? Look what you tackled within yourself. Just amazing. You should be feeling a lot lighter now and freer in yourself. Go take a seat on the banks and dry off and put your socks and shoes back on.

Feel the beauty of this place and call out to a wild animal spirit guide to come forward to meet you and give you a supportive message about your future. Who do you sense? Who do you see? What have they to share with you? Give your thanks and give your gift to this creature and bless the river and roadblocks of rocks for all the lessons you have learnt today. Spray the river now and say thank you. It's time to leave.

Bringing Yourself Back into Your Physical Body

It's time to return. See the physical you, standing there, arms wide open welcoming you back with a big smile. Walk towards your physical self and go around the back of you. Step into your physical body one leg at a time, like a hand slipping back into a glove. One arm, then your other arm. Bring your torso back into the body and head.

Instantly you are transported back into your room and chair. Feel the weight on your shoulders and your feet grounding you. Sense your spirit fully back and present in your body. Take some really deep breaths again; in through your mouth and out through your mouth into the lower abdomen. Now take two or three in through your nose and out through your mouth. Feel yourself in your chair now.

Grounding/Anchoring Yourself and Golden Bubble of Protection

Sense golden roots coming out of your feet and grounding you on the most beautiful earth. Feel it. Sense a golden bubble all around your aura; it is like extra skin—a layer of protection. It is strong and pliable but impenetrable. Feel it. This golden bubble will be activated indefinitely to protect your energy from negative people or anything environmental. Smile. Take a moment just to say thank you to your body. Your heart, your mind, your soul. Finally, open your eyes whenever you feel ready.

Review

Feel renewed; feel at peace, present and joyful. Take notes in your diary— you can read back and reflect on it all when you need to. If you are meditating in a group then allow each person the opportunity to share what magic they have experienced, remembering all the good moments. What did you feel, see, sense, or just know? What lessons can you take away from this that will help you in any way with your beautiful life journey? Feel touched and blessed. Smile.

Chapter Thirty-One
White Buffalo Calf Woman

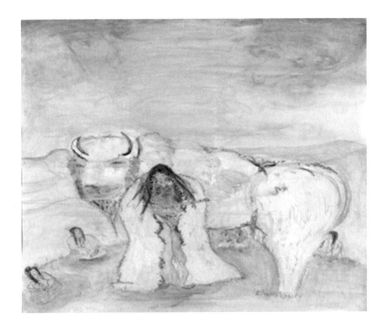

Meet the Native Lakota Indian's Goddess and connect with the Sacred Bundles or gifts, she bestows upon you. This Meditation is about a remembrance of these peoples and their ways, and how to reconnect with the sacred in the landscape.

[Begin your routine first.]

This is a shamanic journey that I will lead you on. Imagine arriving in an open prairie, skirted by a meandering river that seems to cradle and hug an Indian settlement close to it. Can you see it?

Shortly, you are going to meet White Buffalo Calf Woman. The prophecy goes that she brought a Sacred Bundle along with her peace pipe to these people over two thousand years ago. A beautiful woman in white buffalo fur was seen embodied within a white buffalo calf and hence why this Goddess Mother received her name.

Go and mingle amongst the tribal women, medicine women and wise elders of the village. Feel part of the land as they do and feel the inter-connectedness of the community. On you go and enjoy this experience for as long as you like.

Observe the weaving and cooking going on in the settlement, the warriors attending to their horses, the children playing and dogs running around the tepees having fun, chased by the children. Feel the essence of the land risen in this place and how special it feels.

You sense a stirring of the tribal elders, the medicine women and see the female 'Truth Holder' (she holds the essence of the truth of the tribe and its history, no matter what trouble arrives at their door, no matter what war or frictions happen out with or within the tribe). Please do go and take a seat on the grass in the large forming circle, amongst the wise ones. Feel the energy build as everyone sits quietly now legs crossed with hands in lap, in a meditative state.

The Medicine Women Elder stands up and begins to share about who they are all about to meet. She tells about White Buffalo Calf Woman and how she will be appearing from the heavens shortly and offering seven sacred bundles—a gift to her people and to you.

You feel the weight of a bull calf's presence, as this white buffalo calf is witnessed in the light above and growing stronger and brighter as it descends and lands in the middle of the circle. You see the form of a radiant, middle-aged beaded lady superimposed in the body of the calf. Her form begins to grow and you see the white calfskin over her shoulders running down to her feet. You observe her black eyes, the black pleated hair and rosy lips. She is a sight to behold. Everyone feels her energy so powerfully in this circle. Can you? Each bow to her and smile.

She steps away from the bulk of the calf and holds out several items in her hands. White Buffalo Calf Woman smiles and bows to each person, takes a seat and begins to breathe deeper. It seems to raise her vibration and her essence becomes stronger. She talks about the seven sacred bundles.

The first one is the peace pipe. She lights an ornate wooden pipe in her hands and passes it to the Chief. He smokes it and passes it on. This ritual is part of an important unification of the tribe, where each member is equal and each shares in these sacred medicinal herbs within the pipe.

The next ceremony is a purification ritual to cleanse and heal your body and soul, which takes place in a Sweat Lodge. She describes how the ritual really leads you deep into yourself, to be absorbed into the womb of the dark earth as you sit in the blackened out warm tepee. She shares the tale about the naming ceremony and why it is important to share in the energy of this rite for new-born babies. She shares about an adoption rite and a marriage ceremony.

She begins to ask each person to decide what they wish to choose to participate in for the last of the ceremonies. The choices she gives are either a celebratory Sundance around this circle or to go on a private Vision Quest. Or perhaps one to connect with deceased loved ones, or to ask for inspiration from Great Spirit, Creator—this is a celebratory thanksgiving time. What do you choose to experience?

Do your thing and join those who are dancing if you wish, or go sit in solitude on the hill close by and take time to go within and do your own little Vision Quest. Everyone is finished and goes back to sit in their place in the circle once again. Before White Buffalo Calf Women leaves and returns to the heavens, each person has an audience with her. Wait your turn and go within. What would you like to ask her advice on?

Now go and speak directly to White Buffalo Calf Woman, she is awaiting you. Bow, smile and speak to her about your needs and desires and for inspiration from this Mother God Deity. Feel her light and wisdom and power surround you. Feel her presence so loving and so close. Enjoy your time with her for as long as it takes.

Bow and give thanks at the end and offer her your own sacred bundle from your pockets. A love heart pendant she can wear and the blessing of the New Earth holy elixir. She is so delighted with your gifts you can feel her smile fill all of your body in a huge glow of love. Feel it.

She bows, smiles and you go and step away from her, as she looks to everyone for one last time today. Slowly she then begins to merge into the gorgeous baby buffalo, which begins to rise into the sky becoming fainter as they rise.

You all begin to stand and disperse, and you turn to leave the circle and see your own flesh body. The physical you, standing there.

Bringing Yourself Back into Your Physical Body

It's time to return. See the physical you, standing there, arms wide open welcoming you back with a big smile. Walk towards your physical self and go around the back of you. Step into your physical body one leg at a time, like a hand slipping back into a glove. One arm, then your other arm. Bring your torso back into the body and head.

Instantly you are transported back into your room and chair. Feel the weight on your shoulders and your feet grounding you. Sense your spirit fully back and present in your body. Take some really deep breaths again; in through your mouth and out through your mouth into the lower abdomen. Now take two or three in through your nose and out through your mouth. Feel yourself in your chair now.

Grounding/Anchoring Yourself and Golden Bubble of Protection

Sense golden roots coming out of your feet and grounding you on the most beautiful earth. Feel it. Sense a golden bubble all around your aura; it is like extra skin—a layer of protection. It is strong and pliable but impenetrable. Feel it. This golden bubble will be activated indefinitely to protect your energy from negative people or anything environmental. Smile. Take a moment just to say thank you to your body. Your heart, your mind, your soul. Finally, open your eyes whenever you feel ready.

Review

Feel renewed; feel at peace, present and joyful. Take notes in your diary— you can read back and reflect on it all when you need to. If you are meditating in a group then allow each person the opportunity to share what magic they have experienced, remembering all the good moments. What did you feel, see, sense, or just know? What lessons can you take away from this that will help you in any way with your beautiful life journey? Feel touched and blessed. Smile.

Chapter Thirty-Two
Vision Quest

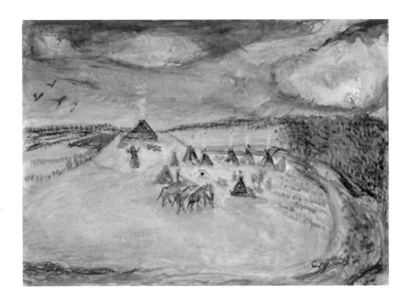

Although quite often thought of as only connected to the Native American Indians, many diverse cultures have taken on a Vision Quest for millennia in search of enlightenment. Buddha sought illumination in 500 BC. When the Buddha fasted in a forest underneath the Bodhi tree the knowledge he gained from this affected the course of history for Buddhism. Jesus went for forty days into the wilderness on his own profound Vision Quest.

He was tempted during this challenging time but overcame his challenges through fasting and communing with the Creator. This Vision Quest you are about to go on will bring you some insights into things you fear and things you can overcome. This will be a meditation to help your growth and enable you to perhaps stretch yourself.

[Begin with your routine.]

Join me on this Shamanic rite of passage, this beautiful journey to the prairie land of the Lakota Native American Indians, and to their settlement by the river. Feel your feet on the land and connect as they do with the living landscape, the breathing land and oxygen-filled sky. See the bison grazing close to the forest, way off to the left of you. There are antelope off in the distance too and you see eagles overhead. How do you feel to be here?

Head to the village, where you will feel the energy of the tribe mingling around the fire pits. Take in the community baking bread and telling stories; see the children playing tag and the Elders talking in a small circle off to the right, close to the riverbed. The braves are tending to their animals and life feels so peaceful and happy. Connect with a wave and smile as you pass through, heading to the mound at the other end of the village, which you spot has an ornate large tepee on top. This is where you will do your personal Vision Quest. Head for it.

Look at the Wise Woman, known as 'Truth-Keeper', she is beckoning you to go up that hill and join her. She is a Shamenka Elder and Healer. Smile and bow as you climb the hill and meet her face-to-face. You both sit outside the tepee's narrow, low entrance. She shares with you the details of what this Sweat Lodge is about. She informs you that you will be having a purification rite as well as a Vision Quest.

She then shows you that the willow sticks that were made to construct this tepee are orientated a foot apart, in honour of the four directions: North, South, East and West. The door of the Lodge is facing west. A pit inside is fourteen feet West of the door and is lined in a semi-circle on the West-side of the fire pit so it is like a reflector. This mound reflects firelight back towards the Sweat Lodge.

Both the fire and pit are masculine in nature. The Sweat Lodge is the feminine principle. The Wise Woman explains the construction of the cedar wooden blocks that are on the fire pit, which honour the four directions again. A block is also included in honour of the above, below and one is also in honour of the Sweat Lodge builder.

Now it's time to enter. Get down on all fours and crawl inside into the dark womb of the sanctuary. It has the fire burning bright. There are cushions and blankets set all around the fire pit. Go take your seat and sit cross-legged, facing the fire.

The Shamenka has joined you and now lays eighteen small rocks on top of the wood. You can see that mist and vapour is beginning to rise from the fire, as the Shamenka pours water onto the rocks. You both breathe in the moisture deep into your lungs. In and out through your mouth. In and out. Feel the steam and the fire rise and fill the whole place. How does it feel in this pitch darkness?

Let go, surrender and allow your Higher Self to guide you into a deeper state of consciousness. Breathe and relax, breathe and relax; deeper and deeper you slip into an altered consciousness. It's glorious and still. See what symbols appear in your vision, notice what pictures form in your mind and which feelings and words come through to you in this state. Stay in this place for as long as you are getting visions and information coming through.

When it is time, begin to take some deeper breaths once again, in through your nose this time and out through your mouth, bringing oxygen into your mind. You are bringing your awareness back into your body and surroundings as you sit here with your eyes now open.

You look into the Shamenka's eyes and you both smile at one another. She reaches over to you with a little gift in her hands—it's a keepsake for you. Give your thanks and offer her a love heart crystal pendant as your offering of thanks and ask if you can spray her and the Sweat Lodge with the New Earth holy water. She nods with a huge humble smile. Do your thing and when complete follow the Shamenka out of the Lodge on your hands and knees. You will see the physical you standing there, waiting on you to take you back home.

Bringing Yourself Back into Your Physical Body

It's time to return. See the physical you, standing there, arms wide open welcoming you back with a big smile. Walk towards your physical self and go around the back of you. Step into your physical body one leg at a time, like a hand slipping back into a glove. One arm, then your other arm. Bring your torso back into the body and head.

Instantly you are transported back into your room and chair. Feel the weight on your shoulders and your feet grounding you. Sense your spirit fully back and present in your body. Take some really deep breaths again; in through your mouth and out through your mouth into the lower abdomen. Now take two or three in through your nose and out through your mouth. Feel yourself in your chair now.

Grounding/Anchoring Yourself and Golden Bubble of Protection

Sense golden roots coming out of your feet and grounding you on the most beautiful earth. Feel it. Sense a golden bubble all around your aura; it is like extra skin—a layer of protection. It is strong and pliable but impenetrable. Feel it. This golden bubble will be activated indefinitely to protect your energy from negative people or anything environmental. Smile. Take a moment just to say thank you to your body. Your heart, your mind, your soul. Finally, open your eyes whenever you feel ready.

Review

Feel renewed; feel at peace, present and joyful. Take notes in your diary— you can read back and reflect on it all when you need to. If you are meditating in a group then allow each person the opportunity to share what magic they have experienced, remembering all the good moments. What did you feel, see, sense, or just know? What lessons can you take away from this that will help you in any way with your beautiful life journey? Feel touched and blessed. Smile.

Chapter Thirty-Three
Market Garden Mother's Larder!

This is a working meditation that takes you into a divine, small allotment in the countryside. There are many varieties of flowering trees, plants and lovely herbs; many that are medicinal. You are going to be guided by the subtle elements of the plants and trees, to pick what would be helpful to you in your life right now. You may need to do your own online research to understand what the medicinal, healing or therapeutic properties are of what you pick, however, in advance—here is some to get you going.

__Common plants__: Potatoes are just full of fibre and potassium and Vitamin C and B6, garlic is amazing for helping common colds, lowering cholesterol levels. Cabbage, full of Vitamin C, plus lowers cholesterol; beetroot is full of fibre, magnesium, iron and potassium, spinach, full of Vitamin C, K and A and is great for eye health. Tomatoes are full of Vitamin C and K and help fight cancers and heart disease. Spring onions or any onions are great for flue's or chest infections and lung issues. Research these ones yourself: Lettuce, sage, celery, avocado, beans, asparagus, mint, sweet pea, corn flour, dandelion, nettles, strawberries, raspberries, blueberries and grapes.

__Medicinal Plant Medicine__ – St John's Wart and Mother's Wart are great for anxiety, low mood, depression and heart issues. Holy Basil for joint pain, inflammation and arthritis. Turmeric is an antioxidant and helps with arthritis and heart issues. Evening Primrose oil is great for skin issues, arthritis and the change of life for women. Lavender and chamomile plants are great calming sedatives for sleep but also lower anxiety. Tea Tree oil is an antiseptic plant that helps with wound healing. Echinacea is a healer and fights the flu plus helps lower blood sugar levels and blood pressure. Ginseng boosts the immune *system and can help increase energy levels. Gingko is great for brain health. Bergamot is useful to reduce inflammation, it is anti-inflammatory and helps with painful cysts, pimples and spots.*

*   ***Fruit Tree Medicine** – Apples and pears are great for gut health, oranges are full of Vitamin C, lemon and lime are good for the skin and lemon for hydration and weight loss. Coconut is great for bone health. It is also an antioxidant. It is rich in copper and iron too.*

*   *Why not investigate what the maple, olive, cherry banana and pomegranate fruits can help you with.*

Settling Down and Breathwork

Get comfortable in your chair, take a deep breath and let it out, shut your eyes now and breathe. In through your mouth, out through your mouth and into your lower abdomen. Deep rhythmic, yogic breaths. Do five of these now; Feeling your head, neck and shoulders begin to drop and relax and your chest and back. Take a couple of nice breaths in through your nose next to five exhaling out through your mouth. Feel your stomach and abdomen hips and whole pelvic girdle relax, feel yourself just melting into the chair. Your thighs, knees, calves and feet are softening and relaxing. How good it feels. Keep your eyes shut throughout the whole guided meditation, it helps you focus within.

Connecting with Mother/Father God or Great Spirit

Now tilt your head upwards and with your eyes shut, use your inner vision to see and connect with the light of Creation, Great Spirit, Mother/Father God—whatever you may call this Light and loving consciousness. Sense an outpouring, down-pouring of beautiful pearlescent light, gently spilling down towards you through cosmos, universe and galaxy into our galaxy and atmosphere. Sense your head tingling in response and the top of your crown opening up to receive this beautiful light. Smile in gratitude to this pure, loving light as it soaks and saturates over your whole aura and through your mind and body.

Smile. Feel it. How good it feels. Feeling the connection to the rest of creation is good. Feel the light pouring down your legs and out the bottom of your feet, into the very core and heart of our beautiful planet. Imagine yourself as a vessel a conduit that is connecting the heavens with our beautiful pristine

Earth. Send a puff of love down into the centre of the Earth and take a moment just to say thank you. Thank you for the shelter, abundance, protection, nourishment and beauty we receive every day. Thank you. Now send a puff of love up to the Great Spirit, all love of creation, for the unseen subtle guidance we receive every day keeping us on track. Give thanks for the Spirit that we are and that we are also part of the Creator or Great Spirit. Thank you.

Pillar of Light

If you are in a circle with others, then visualise a pillar of light, See it shimmering as it descends from the Cosmos, from Great Spirit. Opalescent, quintessence light. Beautiful. Add anyone you wish to step into the pillar of light now, for love support or healing. Remember, it must be in accordance with their own divine will to receive it. This is a universal law. If someone wishes to have their challenging experience it is their choice.

Light Body

Step out of your dense physical body now, which is a light-body—a mirror of yourself. I will guide you safely back at the very end of the journey and ground and anchor you safely. I will also Protect your aura. It's safe to journey with me.

You see in front of you a small but well maintained, hedged allotment. This is your heavenly market garden, full of all the goodness nature can provide. It is a global garden allotment. This means that no matter where the tree or plant comes from, it will be made available to you here now if it is something that any system in your body needs.

Go through the small willow gate and into your magical, colourful market garden. You see a water tap and sparkling yellow hose on a roll-out machine, for watering the trees and plants. It's a fun job you can do as we go through the garden up the rows of this magical allotment.

Firstly, you will take a look at the small bushy plants in rows close to the ground and the spikey-like leafy ones, the bulbous ones and the bushy ones. Have a look at the wispy herbs and tall stalk plants, with big huge heavy leaves around them. You may see an incredible variety of fruit or medicinal trees such as eucalyptus, coconut, apple, pear, orange or olive trees, nut trees, or just sweet-smelling ones. What do you see as you look up the earthy rows and along the rear hedge? I want you to silently converse with the species of trees

148

and plants as you go. Ask them to guide you and communicate with you. Request that they give you little messages as you stop and pick them.

This is your time, so take the little willow basket with you and your spade and go enjoy. Wander up and down the rows of this magical place; look at the colours of the trees off to the left of the garden. You see coconut, cherry, apple, pear, olive, maple, ginkgo, lemon and lime, plum and orange trees. It is truly a sight to behold. Look at them all and the exquisite colour and energy they are sending out to you.

Feel it. You can go to them in a while. Firstly, you must walk up the rows and into the medicinal enclosed part of the garden. You may discover that you are drawn to the apple and pear trees, and wish to communicate with their spirit and get information connected to your gut health. It may be the lime and lemon trees that wish to connect with you, to do with your skin and hydration issues, or even weight loss with the lemon tree. Or the ginkgo tree to help you with the whole spectrum of brain functioning.

This is the new earth's larder and you have been given the abundance of the world, feel the deep blessing of this experience. You will get to taste it all later when you research and make something of the ingredients. There is a thought. You just may learn something new about a particular herb just now though, as you wander up and down the vegetable rows and get down low to smell them— communicate with them as you go. I recommend you look at the herbs too and ask the elemental essence of the herb to communicate with you. On you go.

The first two rows have potatoes, then garlic, which is good for common colds and cholesterol levels. Cabbage is there full of Vitamin C; spring onions, which helps with respiratory issues, then beetroot, which is a great source of fibre, magnesium, iron and potassium. Spinach is an excellent source of Vitamin C, K and A and is great for eye health. Look at the plants and the richness of them all.

How large and healthy the leaves are, and the stalks. Is there any that are flowering? What colour are the petals? Take your hose, remember; the water is turned on. Know there are four settings to work with besides off. One setting is a large shower head type wide spray for more coverage and the lighter spray is for the saplings that are under the white netting tunnels. You can see them in the third row, close to the trees.

There is a very powerful focused jet for established plants with thick stalks and roots to get right in at the root and earth around them, plus a softer jet for more delicate plants. Have fun watering them all as you get into a rhythm. It is a great form of walking meditation. Enjoy. Remember to stop and connect with the elemental nature of the plant. Ask questions, wait for answers in your mind. They will work through telepathy. See the white netted tunnels; make sure to hose the saplings in there.

At the next row, you see the rosemary herbs, little bushes with its spikey-like, stalky leaves. Kneel down by one and smile at the plant. This medicinal herb originates from the Mediterranean and is used in all sorts of lovely culinary dishes to enhance the flavour. It has even been used to ease muscle pain by the Romans in ancient times and boost the circulatory and immune systems. It helps with neurological things in the brain, and it is an anti-ageing ally.

Rosemary improves your digestion and is anti-inflammatory and an antioxidant also. How amazing right? Ask it to communicate with you. It will show you an image, how robust it looks and how inspiring to know of its incredible properties, right? Ok, thank the herb and ask permission to take a cutting for your basket. Move up the row where you see lovely pinkie flower heads on long strong stalks.

It is the turmeric, the wonder spice. Remember you can grow anything from any country in this heavenly healing allotment. It is native to India and we all enjoy a curry with turmeric in it, right? Like Rosemary, turmeric is an anti-oxidant and anti-inflammatory spice and is used in food but is also linked to brain function. Again, go down low and smile sending love to the plant and ask to connect with it and to take a cutting before you move on. Give your thanks and move on up the row, to the holy basil just ahead.

It looks so green and has an abundance of thin rounded healthy leaves on the small bushy plant. It is amazing for treating a fever or common cold, for its amazing healing properties, aiding with respiratory disorders—just as the common onion is when put on the chest like a poultice. This all-round healer helps with children's ailments, tooth or mouth pain, headaches, eye disorders etc. Go communicate through your mind and heart with this holy one. Smile and give your thanks.

Ask if you can take a bunch of it. Time to move on to the next row and you see a large spikey bush of stinging nettles. Don't be afraid of it. Go and kneel beside it. You can make a great brew from it and this stingy one helps with many things including fatigue and arthritic pain. Nettle also helps to eliminate stones from the kidneys and gallbladder, and it is amazing at relieving or lowering systolic blood pressure and relieves tension and stress on your cardiovascular system.

Ask it how you can work with it and take a bunch? Finally, you go take a look at the pale lavender and purple flowering St John's Wart and Mother Wart plants. These are helpful for depression or anxiety, plus heart issues, in the case of Mother Wart. Are the plants all well-watered now?

How was that? Have you filled your basket yet? What trees have drawn you? What do they look like? What draws you? Go over and say your hello, water them all and connect. This is your time. Enjoy.

There is a prayer tree with coloured ribbons way up at the back, almost hidden. Go to it and sit under that beautiful oak tree and write some positive affirmations on the ribbons with the marker pen there. You can even go climb a tree if you fancy after you have finished.

Was that fun? It is time to bless the plants, herbs, flowers and trees with the sacred, magical elixir, the New Earth holy water. This New Eden elixir is imbued into your hose. Know that you can reach each plant and tree, as this is a magical hose. Take a minute to do it. Smile. Wynd the hose back in now; coil it up on the hoe, make sure the tap is off and no drips escape. How satisfying was that?

You have many gifts and you have blessed your garden with a good drink. There is one final thing to do before you leave with your produce. Send out a huge puff of love over the whole of the allotment. Say thank you. Mean it. Time to leave this incredible place. Feel how good life is for you and how abundant you really are. Remember what you have discovered and research anything you are unfamiliar with. You walk out of the garden now and you see yourself.

Bringing Yourself Back into Your Physical Body

It's time to return. See the physical you, standing there, arms wide open welcoming you back with a big smile. Walk towards your physical self and go around the back of you. Step into your physical body one leg at a time, like a hand slipping back into a glove. One arm, then your other arm. Bring your torso back into the body and head.

Instantly you are transported back into your room and chair. Feel the weight on your shoulders and your feet grounding you. Sense your spirit fully back and present in your body. Take some really deep breaths again; in through your mouth and out through your mouth into the lower abdomen. Now take two or three in through your nose and out through your mouth. Feel yourself in your chair now.

Grounding/Anchoring Yourself and Golden Bubble of Protection

Sense golden roots coming out of your feet and grounding you on the most beautiful earth. Feel it. Sense a golden bubble all around your aura; it is like extra skin—a layer of protection. It is strong and pliable but impenetrable. Feel it. This golden bubble will be activated indefinitely to protect your energy from negative people or anything environmental. Smile. Take a moment just to say thank you to your body. Your heart, your mind, your soul. Finally, open your eyes whenever you feel ready.

Review

Feel renewed; feel at peace, present and joyful. Take notes in your diary—you can read back and reflect on it all when you need to. If you are meditating in a group then allow each person the opportunity to share what magic they have experienced, remembering all the good moments. What did you feel, see, sense, or just know? What lessons can you take away from this that will help you in any way with your beautiful life journey? Feel touched and blessed. Smile.

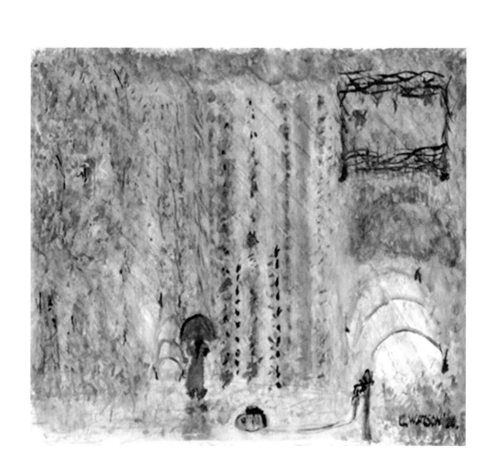

Chapter Thirty-Four
Meeting Queen and Saint
Margaret of Scotland at St
Margaret's Grotto

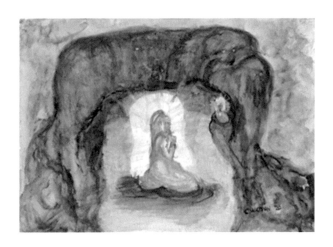

I would like to take you back in time, from the past thousand years of Scottish history to the year 1050. King Malcolm Canmore III ruled the land, with his beautiful, kind, spiritual Beloved Consort and wife, Queen Margaret. It is Margaret, Queen of Scotland that I want to introduce you to. I do hope you make a beautiful and healing connection with her in her grotto/cave.

Firstly, I want to share a little more about Margaret. It was she who reignited Christianity in Scotland and helped deepen the connection between Scotland and the European Courts. Margaret was a very holy Queen; she helped the poor of the land as much as she could and would feed many children at the castle gates before she would eat her own breakfast each morning. Margaret is the only Sainted Queen of Scotland and indeed the whole of the British Isles.

There are remnants of her still to this day, with an Edinburgh school and University being named after her. She also instigated the creation of a safe passage for pilgrims travelling to and from St Andrews town and other sacred sites with the installation of a ferry passage at North and South Queensferry. Her participation in the project is the reason why this passage across the sea was named 'Queens' ferry, in her honour.

These ferries would connect the Old Kingdom of Fife in Scotland, to the new Kingdom of Lothian and Edinburgh: its modern capital. Queen Margaret and Malcolm also blessed Scotland with eight children—four became subsequent Kings of this land. One son became a renowned Bishop, and their daughter married into the French Royal Courts.

To meet Margaret, you will need to go back in time to when the ferries were installed, back thousand years. However, firstly, you need to get yourself settled and ready to journey. Shall we begin?

Imagine yourself going back a thousand years in time, where you have stepped out onto the foreshore of South Queensferry in Scotland, as you see the ferry boat moored and ready to receive you onto it. Step aboard and settle down. The ferry takes off heading for Dunfermline where the Cave is nestled in the valley by the river there. Enjoy the journey.

You arrive at the other side of the Forth estuary and prepare now for your pilgrimage to meet St Margaret by the entrance to her cave, in the valley by the river. As you walk on the land you feel the medieval timeframe you have stepped back into. You may see smoke from cottages and shacks as you go walking now into the valley. Follow the river and tree line, which will guide you as you walk.

Ahead on the left, you see a very humble beautiful young woman standing by a very large cave opening. Prepare yourself mentally and emotionally for meeting this Great Queen and Saint. Send a puff of love from your heart out to Margaret and ask to connect with her. Do this now. Smile.

Know that you have been summoned to go to her as she smiles and waves to you. Know you have a lovely crystal love heart as a gift for her at the end of the meditation and the new earth holy water to give her also. On you go, feel her beautiful energy. It is subtle but full of light and wisdom. You can sense Margaret is in this world but not of it. You can feel her foot in two worlds; the world of spirit and the world of physicality. She is a magical person and your whole spirit feels ignited and enlivened through connecting with her energy.

On you go and bow to her when you come face-to-face. Margaret smiles at you and bows to you and opens up her arm to usher you into the cave. It is lit with candles and has a ledge seat inside it and a small altar that is naturally part of the cave. The ledge seating has cushions—go take a seat beside Saint Margaret. She takes your hand if you feel comfortable with this.

She asks how she can help you in your life today. Share anything that is in your heart, she will listen and give you her wisdom. Enjoy. Offer her your crystal and the elixir, which she takes and thanks you with a smile, and then bows. She asks that you both sit and meditate together and that you allow the cave-like womb, this grotto to heighten the connection to heaven and to the Great Spirit, especially the Divine Mother Aspect of Source.

How did that feel? How wonderful to sit with Margaret like this and feel the connection with her and Spirit. How blessed you feel. Thank Margaret as you both stand up and she leads you to the grotto altar. She places your crystal on the altar and sprays the altar with the new earth elixir. She asks you to also spray her before you leave.

Do this now. She bows to you and you feel the essence of the holy water fizzing all around the altar and Saint Margaret. Feel it yourself. Touch the cave wall, as you say your farewell, leaving Margaret in the grotto to pray.

It is time to head for home now.

Bringing Yourself Back into Your Physical Body

It's time to return. See the physical you, standing there, arms wide open welcoming you back with a big smile. Walk towards your physical self and go around the back of you. Step into your physical body one leg at a time, like a hand slipping back into a glove. One arm, then your other arm. Bring your torso back into the body and head.

Instantly you are transported back into your room and chair. Feel the weight on your shoulders and your feet grounding you. Sense your spirit fully back and present in your body. Take some really deep breaths again; in through your mouth and out through your mouth into the lower abdomen. Now take two or three in through your nose and out through your mouth. Feel yourself in your chair now.

Grounding/Anchoring Yourself and Golden Bubble of Protection

Sense golden roots coming out of your feet and grounding you on the most beautiful earth. Feel it. Sense a golden bubble all around your aura; it is like extra skin—a layer of protection. It is strong and pliable but impenetrable. Feel it. This golden bubble will be activated indefinitely to protect your energy from negative people or anything environmental. Smile. Take a moment just to say thank you to your body. Your heart, your mind, your soul. Finally, open your eyes whenever you feel ready.

Review

Feel renewed; feel at peace, present and joyful. Take notes in your diary—you can read back and reflect on it all when you need to. If you are meditating in a group then allow each person the opportunity to share what magic they have experienced, remembering all the good moments. What did you feel, see, sense, or just know? What lessons can you take away from this that will help you in any way with your beautiful life journey? Feel touched and blessed. Smile.

Chapter Thirty-Five
Personal Mandal

"The flowers perfume has no form, but it pervades space. Likewise, through a spiral of mandalas, formless reality is known."
"Each person's life is like a mandala—a vast, limitless circle. And everything we see, hear and think forms the mandala of our life."
– Anonymous

The meaning of 'mandala' in Sanskrit is a circle. It is used in Hinduism and Buddhism as a sacred special circle. It is a representation of the Galaxy, Universe, Cosmos, as a symbol of life never-ending and where everything is connected to the next thing. We are all connected to one another through subtle cords or strings of energy, like the umbilical or silver cord, especially strong to those we are in relationships with; be it, family or friends.

You are going to work with all of your senses to do a personal, enriching mandala about your journey to this point. Your evolving spirit. You want to see and see it illuminated in heavenly colours, large and awesome, it should lead you into the centre of the circle to the point in the very middle of Creation. You want to feel, touch, smell and taste your mandala.

Imagine what that would be like. Is it sweet as nectar? You should draw what you see in Mediation after this session, so get a pad and coloured felt pens to do this and have it by your side to go straight into when you come back around. Bring your Inner Child along with you, let her or him really participate in this one and bring your sense of deep wonder too. Shall we?

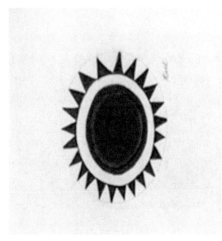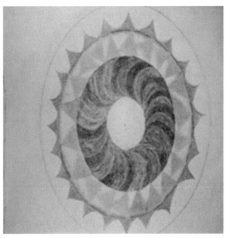

Artwork by Kath Barr Artwork by Kareen Mc Queen

[Begin with your routine.]

Stepping out for your physical body into your mirror body, the light body, you enter into a descending corridor or tunnel well-lit by dancing violet, lavender and white wall torches. It is very dark and very mysterious as you walk down the sloping stone tunnel. You are going to enter into the master artists hermits cave. She is You, she is your unconscious mind and Divine Soul-self waiting to meet you and settle you down in her womb like a warm dark cave. Stone walls encase you down there, which is nurturing and comforting, a homecoming of sorts.

It is very cosy as there are thick feather-down blankets on the floor and pillows to lie down on and snuggle under. How do you feel? Bring your Inner Child into your present journey. Feel the wonder and excitement build. The cave is filled with essential oils, the most sacred aromas of all time. They will help induce you into a very deep space, where you are so alive in yourself and able to view the scene that is going to happen on the ceiling of the cave.

You see an opening appear in the stone and a violet hazy light flooding out—feel the loving energy in this light as you are thrilled to go in and meet your master self. The Creator of you. See ahead, can you see yourself, the Artist? She or he has been expecting you, on you go. Bow and say your hellos. Hug. She leads you to the centre of the dark cave, again it is lit around the floor in soft up-lights, which help you see where you are going. It looks so comfortable and inviting, as does the big soft thick blankets and pillows.

She asks you to go lie down and breathe again in through your nose and out through your mouth this time. Bringing oxygen into your mind, your third eye, the all-seeing inner eye. All the lights are dimmed and fade out. You are in a total blackout but it feels so alive and sensory. Mother's Womb. The womb of all potential. Feel it smile.

Ask your higher self and soul self to help you illuminate, as you begin to create and form the start of your own personal mandala. This mandala will represent how you feel at this place in your life, how illuminated and inter-connected you feel to your own self, your own soul and to others. The colours will reflect your mood, your energy, your creativity, your sparkle, your light. Make it incredible. Make it powerful and special. This is your time.

You will see a brush stroke begin in neon heavenly light on the roof of your cave. Watch and contribute to its creation. Enjoy the feel of all aspects of you working together; your Inner Child, your Inner Male and Female self and your Higher self and Soul self.

Ask your Higher Mind and Higher Heart to interpret what you are seeing as you see it form, build and complete itself. No rush, this is your time, take as long as you like. Make it count. Remember to draw what you see later and keep it as a keepsake.

The lights begin to rise from the ground, bringing your consciousness back more to the present. Hold all the memories of this meditation; the feelings and the colours, as your personal mandala fades too. Your master artist self comes over and helps you to sit up and gather yourself again. She gives you a little keepsake gift, one to remember her or him by.

Remember we always have a gift in a pocket and the new earth essence in the other. So stand up and look at what you were gifted and say your thank you with a bow and a hug. Then give your gifts. It's time to head out of this gorgeous black cave and upwards into your physical space through that long tunnel. Say goodbye and wave as you exit this fabulous place. What gift did she give you?

At the very top of the tunnel you see the physical you, smiling waving, and very, very, happy to see you.

Bringing Yourself Back into Your Physical Body

It's time to return. See the physical you, standing there, arms wide open welcoming you back with a big smile. Walk towards your physical self and go around the back of you. Step into your physical body one leg at a time, like a hand slipping back into a glove. One arm, then your other arm. Bring your torso back into the body and head.

Instantly you are transported back into your room and chair. Feel the weight on your shoulders and your feet grounding you. Sense your spirit fully back and present in your body. Take some really deep breaths again; in through your mouth and out through your mouth into the lower abdomen. Now take two or three in through your nose and out through your mouth. Feel yourself in your chair now.

Grounding/Anchoring Yourself and Golden Bubble of Protection

Sense golden roots coming out of your feet and grounding you on the most beautiful earth. Feel it. Sense a golden bubble all around your aura; it is like extra skin—a layer of protection. It is strong and pliable but impenetrable. Feel it. This golden bubble will be activated indefinitely to protect your energy from negative people or anything environmental. Smile. Take a moment just to say thank you to your body. Your heart, your mind, your soul. Finally, open your eyes whenever you feel ready.

Review

Feel renewed; feel at peace, present and joyful. Take notes in your diary—you can read back and reflect on it all when you need to. If you are meditating in a group then allow each person the opportunity to share what magic they have experienced, remembering all the good moments. What did you feel, see, sense, or just know? What lessons can you take away from this that will help you in any way with your beautiful life journey? Feel touched and blessed. Smile.

Chapter Thirty-Six
Overview of All of the Rainbow
Path Series Meditations

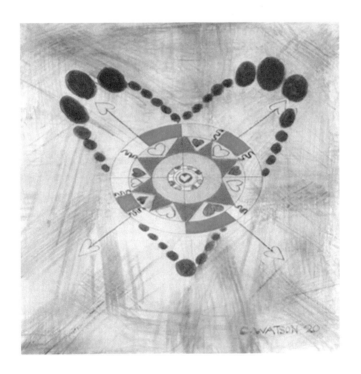

1. Archangel Michael and Foot soldiers (Protection)
2. Archangel Uriel (Communication)
3. Archangel Gabriel (Messenger of the Heart Love/Healing)
4. Archangel Raphael (Healing Journey)
5. Angelic Realm (Meeting all four) Archangels
6. Guardian Angel and Spirit Guide (Heavenly personal) allies
7. Lord Sananda (Cosmic Christ)
8. Mary Magdalene (Christ's Beloved)

9. Quan Yin (Chinese Goddess of Unconditional Love)
10. Lady Paradisia (New Earth Mother)
11. White Buffalo Calf Woman (Lakota Native American Indian Goddess)
12. St Brigid and Ceridwen (Irish Celtic Goddesses. Healing journey)
13. Meeting Spirit of Africa. First Mother (African Mother Goddess) – Mawu
14. ISIS, Egyptian Goddess. (Trip to the Great Pyramid. Initiation in Kings Chamber)
15. Lady Athena (Greek Goddess)
16. Lakshmi Goddess (Asian Lotus Goddess)
17. Freya, The Norse Goddess (Norse power)
18. Margaret, St and Queen of Scotland (Meet in her Cave in Dunfermline)
19. Lady Reshel and Rosslyn Chapel (Keystone activation initiation)
20. Activating the Reshel Grid (multidimensional huge initiation)
21. St Germain and His Torchlight Precession (Initiation by Colour)
22. St Anthony (Meeting at Cave on Arthur Seat)
23. Celtic Round House (Duddingston Loch, Meeting the ancestors)
24. Ascension Seat and Meeting the Dragons (St Anthony's Chapel on Arthur Seat)
25. Life Review and Baptism (Reflective seven hundred and eighty degrees, inside and out)
26. Activating the Vagus Nerve (Deep inner healing work)
27. The Great Pyramid. Meeting Shekhina (Colour healing in Giza)
28. The Gardener (uprooting issues/healing)
29. Rainbow Ribbons (colour healing)
30. Past lives through the Dimensional Doorway (visiting a past time, healing)
31. Past Lives
32. The Robin Redbreast and Meeting Christ (Divine connectedness)
33. Forest of the Olive Heart (Heart Healing)
34. Picturing Your Future – The Journey (Healing/clearing and Manifestation work)
35. Stepping Stones (overcoming life's obstacles)
36. Yin and Yang (Balancing the inner male and inner female)
37. Inner Reflection (reviewing self)
38. Waiting in Heavens Wings (Inner child fun)

39. Healing the Inner Child (healing work)
40. Dolphin and Whales (Deep peace/oceanic connections)
41. Transformation 101 (Initiation)
42. Garden of Eden (Manifesting Future worlds)
43. Illumination (Pineal/hypothalamus/Inner healing work)
44. New Earth – Stargate Opening (cosmic journey)
45. Arthur Seat Activation work (Equinox)
46. Detoxifying the Pineal and activating the third eye (deep psychic cleanse and re-boot)
47. 9 Cosmic Forces (Initiatory)
48. Arkansas Crystal River (crystal initiations)
49. Healing of the sea with Dolphin and Whale Power (Connectedness experience)
50. Native American Indian Regression (Past Lives)
51. Vision Quest (inner Elemental healing)
52. Meet your Animal and Spirit Guide (invisible support)
53. Stairway in The Clouds (releasing issues)
54. Crystal Cave (Feeling the power of crystals)
55. Hawks Nest (Perspective of Bird)
56. Swan Beauty (inner love and appreciation)
57. Meeting Your Power Animal (Guide to support your life journey)
58. The Healing Cabin (beautiful nature journey and Healing) Listen to it on You Tube Listen to it on You Tube https://youtu.be/CFFanuJWxlac
59. Soul Pilgrimage (Acquainting yourself with Soul-Self)
60. Soul Merge (144 Soul Monad connection to our Over-Soul)
61. Meet Your Twin Flame (The other half of your soul)
62. Dancing Your Love Pattern (Create your LIFE MANDALA)
63. The World Tree (Connecting with micro and macro cosmos)
64. Uniting The Galactic, Universal and Cosmic Hearts Cosmic elevated experience)
65. Tree Meditation (Real connection with the spirit of trees)
66. Mawu (Ma Woo) (African Mother Earth Goddess)
67. IXCHEL (Ish-shell) (Mayan Medicine Goddess)
68. Diana Queen of The Pagans (Celtic Nature journey)
69. The Sphinx (Occult Mysteries)
70. The Temple Oasis (Desert journey)

71. Fortingal Yew and Fairy Circle (5,000-year-old Yew connection)
72. Jack and the Beanstalk and the Tree House (Higher perspective on life/world)
73. Manifestation Train (Creating the things you desire)
74. Inner Child (Healing childhood issues)
75. The Cave (going within. Facing fears)
76. Hot Air Balloon (Higher perspective)
77. Making Waves -Message in a Bottle (Connecting to Higher Self)
78. Inner Body Review (Self-Healing)
79. Crop Circles and The Watchers (ethereal guardians)
80. The Pyramid Centre, North Berwick (Visions of a Future World Spiritual Centre)
81. The Labyrinth (Inner quest)
82. The Dragon (ethereal connections)
83. The Horse Whisperer (Equestrian journey in England)
84. The Balm Well (Edinburgh holy well blessings)
85. Rosefield (healing with the red ray)
86. Merlin and the Standing stones (mystical wisdom)
87. Fountain of Youth (replenishing experience)
88. Casting The Net (Hauling in life's gifts and riches)
89. Lions Gate Initiation (Cosmic Initiation)
90. Soaring High (Higher perspective)
91. Wishing Well (Rich Manifestations/blessings)
92. Facing your Shadow (facing the dark side of self)
93. The Holy Trail (Mysticism of the Knights Templar, Mary and Jesus)
94. Crystal Skulls (Crystal skull consciousness/wisdom)
95. Colour Therapy (Healing through colour)
96. The Platinum Ray (Dolphin and Whale healing energy)
97. The Sacred Cove (Gilmerton, Edinburgh) (Scottish mystery school work)
98. Summer Solstice (Sun alignments/world work)
99. Meeting Your Higher Self (The perfected aspect of your being) Kundalini The Flame Within (Initiation of inner firepower).
100. Climbing a Mountain (Facing adversities/overcoming).
101. Standing Stone Circle (reconnecting with the past).
102. The Bonfire (casting out issues/pain).

103. The Butterfly (Transformation, self-alchemy).

104. Dimensions (Step through the dimensional door).

105. Manifesting Abundance (work towards creating all your wealth).

106. Heart Hearth (deep heart work) Listen to an introduction on You Tube https://youtu.be/OgT59N2-g4w

107. 24 Strand DNA Activation (Cellular Activation and healing).

108. Cosmic Mother 11:11 (Connecting through the ocean to Creatrix).

109. Sensuous Lovers, tantric journey (Couple meditation, reconnection) Listen to it on You Tube https://youtu.be/luDX9GmDNb4

110. Venus Temple, tantric technique (Lovers dance then tantric practice).

111. Samye Ling Monastery (Buddhist visit to temple).

112. The Seagull (Higher perspective /choices).

113. Gulliver's Travels (Magic and mystery).

114. The Maize (Inner journeying).

115. Candle Gazing (Beauty and inner flamework).

116. Shiva Ring of Fire (Cosmic flamework).

117. Healing Blood and Lymph (cellular healing).

118. The Zodiac (Working with the elements).

119. Starship Athena and the healing chamber (inter-dimensional connection and healing).

120. Meeting yours 144 Soul Monad (Integrating wholeness).

121. The Seven Rays (balancing all the chakra systems).

122. Breathing Colour (Healing work).

123. Star Alignment (Cosmic connecting).

124. Meeting Lord Ashtar of Ashtar Command (Inter-dimensional contact).

125. Venus – Goddess of Love (Sensual and all-loving).

126. The Butterfly (Transformation)

127. Life Path and Mission (Getting on the right life path).

128. Healing Your Shadow (Healing our darkness. Meeting The Morrigan and Daughters darkness).

129. Road Trip (Manifesting Future).

130. Full Moon Work (Nature honouring).

131. Shifting Paradigm's (Raising consciousness).

132. IONA – The Dove (Sacred journey to Holy Isle).

133. Synergy and Hilary – Two Crystal Skulls (Beloved Twin Flames).

134. 6th Night of the Galactic Underworld (Mayan mysteries).

135. 11:11:11 Alchemy (Inner work)

136. New Earth (Helping raise new conscious earth).

137. Archangel Metatron (Archangel who is Light Keeper).

138. Angelic Guide and Deceased one (Connecting to a deceased loved one).

139. Archangel Chamuel – Treasure at end of the rainbow (Nature journey).

140. Heart Merge (Honouring our Sacred Heart and expanding it).

141. Cat Spirit (Draw from the energy of the Big Cats essence).

142. Heart (Really connecting with heart love).

143. King Arthur and Knights of Round Table (Grail legend work, magic/mystery).

144. Egyptian Nephthys and Anubis (Visiting our Dark Side).

145. Egyptian King – Osiris (Christ Green Man Energy connection).

146. Gracing our Magic. (Meeting aspects of our- selves).

147. Soul Merge (With Divine Mother/Father).

148. The Caduceus. Raphael's Healing Rod (Healing work).

149. Stonehenge. Meeting Archangel Raziel (Magic and mysteries).

150. Flower Within (seeing our own beauty).

151. Pure Relaxation (Working through softening the body).

152. 4th Dimensional Healing (Cellular healing work).

153. 1 Air Element Journey (experience working with this element).

154. Guinevere (Insight and drawing from her presence).

155. Earth Mother – Lady Paradisia (Meet The New Gaia).

156. New Moon in Aries (Moon Magic celebrations).

157. Caduceus (Healing through the kundalini).

158. Alpha and Omega (New Beginnings).

159. Trefuilngid Tre-Oechair, Giant of the Gods (Irish Celtic Tree God).

160. Praying Hands of Mary (Meet Mary Magdalene or Mother Mary on holy mountain).

161. Crystal Gridding on Solstice (New Earthwork).

162. Power Animal and Animal Guides (New Earth helpers).

163. Sacred healing Spa (Meet Quan Yin).

164. Meeting Lord Sananda and Lady Nada (Glastonbury Standing Stones).

165. Mars, The Red Planet (Mysteries).

166. Sacred Super Powerball (Healing work).

167. Fiery Dragon (sensuous).

168. Soul Searching (Connecting with your Soul, insights).

169. Black Panther (Power animal great spirit).

170. Sculptor's Cave, Elgin, Moray (Ancient wisdom and advice).

171. Japanese Geisha and Goddess (Learning about precision/routine, structure).

172. Inner review and healing journey (Deep inner clearing work through body scanning).

173. Violet Cave in Lake Tahoe (Meeting St Germain. Third Eye work and magic).

174. Market Garden (Healing journey through herbs and plant medicine).

175. The Snowball Effect (Overcoming phobias and fears).

YouTube

If you wish to go on a guided journey by yourself, then please go onto the YouTube channel and listen to Heart-Hearth or The Healing Cabin or Sensuous Lovers, Tantric Journey (Introduction).

"Know thy Self"

– A quote by the ancient Greek aphorism, which is one of the Delphic maxims. It is inscribed on the Temple of Apollo.

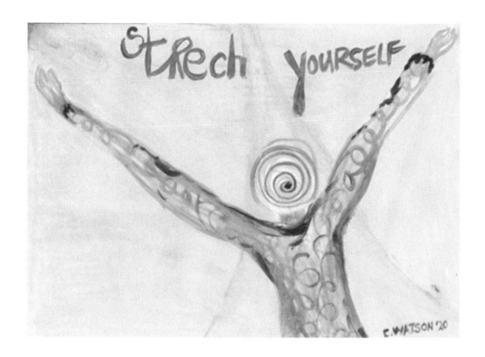

Contact Details:
Email: carolwatson_au@yahoo.com;
Facebook: Rainbow Path 101
or visit www.calmblue.org.uk